MY IMMUNE SYSTEM AND M.S. FIVE YEARS LATER

J.L. WILSON, E.A.

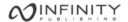

All rights reserved. No part of this book shall be reproduced or transmitted in any form or by any means, electronic, mechanical, magnetic, photographic including photocopying, recording or by any information storage and retrieval system, without prior written permission of the publisher. No patent liability is assumed with respect to the use of the information contained herein. Although every precaution has been taken in the preparation of this book, the publisher and author assume no responsibility for errors or omissions. Neither is any liability assumed for damages resulting from the use of the information contained herein.

Copyright © 2011 by J.L. Wilson, E.A.

ISBN 978-0-7414-6559-7 Hard Cover
ISBN 978-0-7414-6743-0 Paperback
ISBN 978-0-7414-9411-5 eBook

Printed in the United States of America

Published October 2012

INFINITY PUBLISHING
1094 New DeHaven Street, Suite 100
West Conshohocken, PA 19428-2713
Toll-free (877) BUY BOOK
Local Phone (610) 941-9999
Fax (610) 941-9959
Info@buybooksontheweb.com
www.buybooksontheweb.com

CONTENTS

BACKGROUND   1

CHAPTER 1
EXERCISE- LIFESTYLE CHANGE – PHASE ONE   6

CHAPTER 2
NUTRITION-LIFESTYLE CHANGE
PHASES TWO AND THREE   33

CHAPTER 3
SLEEP'S ENORMOUS IMPACT ON LIVING
AND FEELING HEALTHY   59

CHAPTER 4
YOUR OWN STRESS-LESS-NESS GAME PLAN   72

CHAPTER 5
THE RIGHT PERSPECTIVE-ATTITUDE   85

CHAPTER 6
YOU COULD AND NEVER SHOULD TAKE
THIS JOURNEY ALONE   96

CHAPTER 7
TEN YEARS LATER WITH MY LIMP   112

RECOMMENDED READING LIST   130

BACKGROUND
M.S. AND MY IMMUNE SYSTEM
FIVE YEARS LATER

After an overwhelming positive response to my first book on the subject of m.s. (multiple sclerosis), I was encouraged to follow up with a sequel. The research and outline for this book began less than six months after publication of book one.

Verbal reflections included "when are you going to start the second one" to "your book is such a blessing to others with m.s." Medical doctors sought to find me and made prolific comments about book one. "You made the book affordable, it is very needed information" and "how much further along are you?" These comments cemented the nucleus and blueprint to write book two.

All along in writing book one, it was my desire to give others with m.s., a degenerative disease, at least one of the gifts I received. The book also picked up a big following from people who suffer from another degenerative disease, diabetes. I've since learned that this has been primarily because many doctor and expert recommendations to fight m.s. simulate diabetic recommendations.

In book one I sought to share with everyone I could reach in my writing the success of my efforts to rebuild my immune system. Why my Immune system as a topic? Research showed the immune system houses the components that multiple sclerosis launches its attack on. My initial efforts were limited as to my knowledge and resources. Even though I used the services of a leading and reputable publisher, the audience interviewed let me know more could and should be done.

My mission to find and present more core research efforts led me to the professional research teams of Harvard Medical, Cleveland Clinic and Mayo Clinic. Excerpts from much of their work are found in book two. The knowledge scope of this disease (m.s.) and many other degenerative diseases appeared weak to me. Experts have found no cure and do not know the exact cause of m.s.

My vision in book two is to expand areas that book one touched. Many of the expansion ideas came from readers of book one. My inspiration is to share the change for me to good health which remains five and one half years later. Therefore, the task of writing a more comprehensive and larger book was not a secondary worry nor bother.

Lifestyle, consistency, courage and faith are my themes as you journey through my second book on m.s. It is my desire that you will be prompted to visit book one and look at some of the invaluable and reliable resources used to assist me with research and compilation.

The journey living with multiple sclerosis has not at all been regretful nor sad. My initial reaction when first diagnosed was devastation. Quickly, I came to grips with my mission not to let devastation void me. My plan worked or I should better say God's plan for me to get better and remain free of m.s. setbacks and other major diseases worked. Five years later after following an all natural approach and regular doctor visits to my team of medical doctors, I am a pretty "healthy dude," as one of my clients regularly chants.

Today, I continue with this all natural approach. I take no medications for m.s. Only a couple of maintenance medications have been used for overall health and bacterial infection purposes during a five and one half year consecutive span. The prescribing physician has become one of my allies and team doctors. My medical history has not seen me with a cold nor headache during this five and one half year period. In fact, no major illness has surfaced and only a couple of medical flare-up experiences. These flare-ups were treatable and their sources determined not to be linked to m.s.

My walk with m.s. has taught me I am not invincible but somebody bigger than me is responsible for my successes. No way will I credit all of this to my natural approach and team of doctors. God gave me this plan and unwavering faith in God keeps me complete.

Following is a direct quote of some definitive and reliable internet information on the human immune system. This is supplied by the National Institute of Allergy and Infectious Diseases.

IMMUNE SYSTEM

The immune system is a network of cells, tissues, and organs that work together to defend the body against attacks by "foreign" invaders. These are primary microbes- tiny organisms such as bacteria, parasites, and fungi that cause infections. Viruses also cause infections, but are too primitive to be classified as living organisms. The human body provides an ideal environment for many microbes. It is the immune system's job to keep them out or, failing that, to seek out and destroy them.

When the immune system hits the wrong target, however, it can unleash a torrent of disorders, including allergic diseases, arthritis, and form of diabetes. If the immune system is crippled, other kinds of diseases result.

The immune system is amazingly complex. It can recognize and remember millions of different enemies, and it can produce secretions (release of fluids) and cells to match up with and wipe out nearly all of them.

The secret to success is an elaborate and dynamic communications network. Millions and millions of cells, organized into sets and subsets, gather like clouds of bees swarming around a hive and pass information back and forth in response to an infection. Once immune cells receive the alarm, they become activated and begin to produce powerful chemicals. These substances allow the cells to regulate their own growth and behavior, enlist other immune cells, and direct the new recruits to trouble spots.

Although scientists have learned much about the immune system, they continue to study how the body launches attacks that destroy invading microbes, infected cells, and tumors while ignoring healthy tissues. New technologies for identifying individual immune cells are now allowing scientists to determine quickly which targets are triggering an immune response. Improvements in microscopy are permitting the first- ever observations of living B cells, T cells, and other cells as they interact within lymph nodes and other body tissues.

In addition, scientists are rapidly unraveling the genetic blueprints that direct the human immune response, as well as those that dictate the biology of bacteria, viruses, and parasites. The combination of new technology and expanded genetic information will no doubt reveal even more about how the body protects itself from disease.

CHAPTER 1
EXERCISE-LIFESTYLE CHANGE – PHASE ONE

It didn't occur to me until mid 2008 that I had adopted an **exercise lifestyle** change. In one of my favorite gym spots I saw a mutual friend. This friend and I had frequented at least two of the same gym spots for over five years. This time he gave me the traditional embrace and handshake. As he made it to his next workout machine, he said look at you. I tell people all the time it is about lifestyle.

Marsailles comments were centered around the fact that I am at least twenty years older than him but I maintain a consistent and well conditioned fitness routine. This routine shows in my vigor and appearance as he emphasizes. He was amazed at the many times he had regularly seen me in the past three weeks in two different gyms. What was unique about this visit was that it was the second consecutive Saturday we had managed to bump into each other at the same facility. Needless to say comments like that gets you pumping but what is more meaningful to me is that it lets me know I am on the right fitness track.

Lifestyle is defined as a way of life of an individual or group. An internet commentary expands this definition by saying that "a lifestyle is a characteristic bundle of behaviors that make sense to both others and oneself in a given time and place. This includes social relations, consumption, entertainment, and dress. The behaviors and practices within lifestyles are a mixture of habits, conventional ways of doing things, and reasonable actions. A lifestyle typically reflects an individual's attitudes, values or worldview." It took this definition for me to fully grasp the loose use of the term lifestyle in the gym.

Lifestyle change for me in the health and fitness arena consists of different components. One key component is walking daily. My mindset and body feel a strong urge each day to do something health related for me. This mindset keeps me from feeling like I have let my body and inner self down if I don't accomplish my daily fitness goals. Body and memory remind me of the frightful events of the past that pole vaulted me into exercising more vigorously. Some days it is just these tidbit fear thoughts that get me going each day. Most of the times it is just that urge within to do something I thoroughly enjoy.

In past years I was confronted with stumbling and falls while walking normally. Walking was a constant struggle at one point until I continued with exercises targeted at my hamstrings and leg muscles. This increased my quad and leg mass as well as overall leg strength. Walking for exercise began when I recognized this strength and new energy associated with it. Today I continue walking with improvement seen every week. Most noticeable remains lack of stumbling and falling. Now I feel stronger and walk briskly at times. Even a slight run/trot is attempted by me at times.

However, I am not ready to challenge running yet. Mentally, I have not prepared myself. Much relied upon medical research suggests running "reduces disability and may help you live longer." Common sense must apply when it comes to making transitions from the health and fitness circles that have brought me this far.

Mental preparation is needed to calm the fear of moving swiftly without falls. Running is a coordinated effort requiring great leg and hamstring strength to endure.

Stability, endurance and balance are critical factors in achieving successful runs. The leg and hamstring strength have arrived. Strength and endurance are close to where I want them to be but require more stability at length. Multiple sclerosis took its toll on my balance in its early stages. Now, more self-reassurance is required.

My improved balance was the first visible proof to friends and especially to long time clients that I had gotten better. Early on I remember swaying in front of people like an open door with wind blowing and not having anything to break my fall. Many times the person in front of me (particularly men) responded by grasping my shoulder to break my fall. Most of the times I would not completely fall but the swaying gave the person in front of me the appearance I was headed to the floor. Even my barber's son at times had been concerned to the point of helping me to the barber's chair.

My most memorable balance-less moments came at one of my best friend's Christmas parties. My mate was probably the only person at the party who knew of my balance problems. We raced to the dance floor to step to the beat of one of her favorite tunes. We danced over ten minutes to the tune because the dee-jay knew it was one of her favorites. When we went back to our seat another friend and his date had taken their seats at our table.

This friend was still active as one of "Atlanta's finest." Days later after the party, this friend came to my office for an early retirement consultation. He entered my office with his usual humor and blasted me about being tipsy at the party a few days before. He was referring to my after dance walk from the dance floor back to my table and seat. He said my dancing was fine but he noticed me staggering in route from the dance floor to the table. Normal for me, I offered no explanation about my m.s. condition.

Instead my mate and I discussed the event and the party. She laughed so loud and hard until tears came from her eyes. This laughter was because alcohol had been non-existent for me no matter how cheap or free it was. The use of a powerful medication by injection made that more of an exclamation point. Further she said only a policeman at the party openly noticed me going back and forth off the dance floor.

Today staggering and swaying is rare. The memorable moments of my initial stages of walking while stumbling and staggering without any encouragement continue to linger. It is these moments that cause me to delay attempting to run until my balance is better prepared.

Each day I go on my walk without encouragement from a mate, friend or family member. Many days I start inside of my home with floor stretch exercises followed by step board exercises aimed at flexibility of joints and muscles. These exercises get me feeling like I move with greater ease and sense no tightness of muscles. Next the daily walk begins. This walk is no less than three fourth mile each morning. This gets the body juices flowing and the morning air gets my lungs feeling strong giving them good breathing space. As a result I don't feel stuffed up (congested) no matter what season of the year it is. Yes, I walk spring, summer, fall and winter. My body adapts to the temperature change with the season.

Many questions come from people (strangers), acquaintances or friends who notice me walking along my walk route. One of the favorite questions I have come to expect is ("Does the pollen bother you"). My usual reply is, no, it does not. My body yearns for the fresh air daily and it defends off outside elements that would have made me sick over five years ago. My own body has taught me the air is just one critical element it needs daily to make this defensive stand.

My brave walking attempts ballooned a few years ago in year two of my rehab efforts during the fall of the year. As my son continued his participation in monthly 5k and 10k running events this signaled me to begin walking while waiting at the start/finish line. The big test came at his first half marathon run. After waiting so long for his return I had little choice but to walk. When I looked up, amazement set in because I had wondered off farther than planned.

Kevin's half marathon race was my catalyst for walking. Walking continued the full season that year. No kind of allergy nor health condition came upon me that year nor afterwards.

Atlanta fall weather produces great air and a lot of windy conditions most of the time. Many people complain about Georgia's fall weeds (ragweed, example) and pollens from trees and shrubs. In years prior to my walking for health, I experienced sniffles but not the kind of problems I had seen my Atlanta family members encounter. We had everything from puffy eyes, red eyes, to skin irritations in the family. Most of my members had to limit their outside activities during the fall or even wear goggles in certain instances. Fall walks during my five year walk for health have eliminated my sniffles and bad air described by many people.

Some of my most testy m.s. conditions during my early battle arose during winter months. Night sweats and feverish conditions persisted weekly. These five years of maintaining my immune system have caused me to show no signs of the kinds of winter related ill conditions experienced in the past.

Another battle for me in my early years with m.s. was stiff joints mainly in the winter months. Many days I tried to walk leisurely at a comfortable pace but my leg muscles would not cooperate. My moving so slowly was ignored until I overheard a group of gym basketball youngsters taking an outside break as I was leaving. The comments were about "slow motion." That grabbed my attention. You really don't know yourself how fast you are progressing when moving, walking, etc. Outsiders such as those youngster comments are your best gauge. Maintaining my walks for health year round for the last five years has significantly caused my joints, muscles and stiff joints to react with more flexibility.

Stiff joints appeared in articles related to arthritis. One of the most significant articles that grasped my attention was in a special Mayo Clinic report. Mayo's report described two main types of arthritis occurring in more than 100 forms with varying signs and symptoms. It further stated that "generally, arthritis refers to a disease of the joints, which can often result in joint pain, swelling, stiffness- or loss of joint function over time." The two most common types cited were osteoarthritis and rheumatoid arthritis.

Mayo's report stated that osteoarthritis is often called "degenerative or wear-and-tear arthritis. Osteoarthritis usually appears after age 40 or 50 and develops slowly. Rheumatoid arthritis usually begins between ages 25 and 50, often developing within weeks or months. About 75 percent of those with rheumatoid arthritis are women." Prior reading and research of other leading medical publications had indicated that m.s. reacted a lot like arthritis. This signaled me to look at the treatments used for both.

That included physical conditioning as well as nutritional applications. Mayo ended its arthritis report by stating that "you may not be able to make arthritis pain totally go away or do everything you once could. You make the most of what you can do, which includes fully utilizing medical therapies available to you. This includes leading a joint-healthy lifestyle, and maintaining a positive attitude."

My Immune System and M.S. Five Years Later

When I began my winter walks, my greatest fear was catching colds, flu or congestion. Managing to dress in layers of clothing while keeping myself comfortable in Georgia winter conditions was a priority. These walks continued in single digit and teen temperatures during the last five years. This was a huge milestone compared to my past years in Atlanta. My family and I raced for cover and remained indoors as much as possible in past years. This was to avoid the same sort of illnesses I began challenging while walking for health. Recently, I found some neat thermal lined winter tops for severe temperatures. This gear is very comfortable while walking.

Spring walks take me back to sniffle and pollen season months. For me this season brings welcomed fresh air into my lungs and allow me to breathe comfortably. No congestion but free flowing air through my nostrils and lungs persists. Usually, the breezy Atlanta spring temperatures cause me to wear a light top and light athletic shirt underneath but nothing heavyweight.

Summer conditions resemble spring now. This season allows me to take off all tops except a muscle style or light-weight athletic shirt. Choice of other free flowing garments pack my athletic closet for summer walks. The usual hot and humid summer weather conditions of Atlanta never bother me now. In fact, I look forward to these temperatures. My endurance while walking and doing other outside activities has improved from year to year. Aside from endurance, I also experience huge flexibility improvement of my entire body and joints. Early in my dealing with m.s., I encountered two heat related attacks or flare ups (in medical terms). Research showed me this was common in many m.s. cases.

Rarely, scheduling conflicts or sleeping later than normal delays this walk. When this delay happens, I have a backup plan. Usually, it is to walk in the evening when I arrive back home. Sometimes, this doesn't happen and that is why I try hard to stick with the morning schedule.

When I am not traveling for business or pleasure, I usually keep the walk near my home trail. However, I do have backup trails nearby which I frequent. Travel does not keep me from walking nor performing any of my fitness routines. Whenever I book distant travel accommodations, I ask about recommended outside walking spots nearby and conditions. Conditions such as safety, and whether walking is allowed in these areas are two typical concerns. Often times, it is a course around a nearby mall. The key is I get it in and it is not a boresome nor regretful activity.

Harvard Medical has strongly advocated in some of its past medical reports the "vitamins in your legs" are good for your health. There is continuing research to show the effects of dietary supplements versus exercise for heart disease and cancer. Harvard further has stated "regular exercise is a proven way to achieve many of the benefits claimed for vitamins and other supplements., even for people who also eat properly."

Harvard and other leading medical experts have suggested that "insufficient exercise is a major cause of disability and death." Multiple Sclerosis would fall in the disability category. This lack of exercising is linked not only to disability but to four of the leading causes of death in America- heart disease, cancer, stroke, and diabetes in these expert findings. Therefore, strength training exercises are a big component of my health and fitness lifestyle.

My initial research over four years ago showed me that multiple sclerosis has the potential to cause multiple problems. This includes muscle weakness, balance problems, fatigue, visual difficulties, memory loss as well as trouble speaking and depression. In many cases as it progresses, it could cause a disability noticeable from the outside such as the limp in my left leg. Other disabilities may not be so easy to detect but eventually makes its presence either felt or known. It could be detected in the arms, hands, sight or any muscular area of the body.

My mindset remains to combat m.s. head-on by consistently exercising minimum three days per week. This type of activity has assisted in rebuilding all of my body functions to the point that I don't thirst for a walking aid such as a cane or scooter. Instead, I remain highly independent. Remember this exercise is in addition to the other daily things I must do to maintain myself. All of these daily must do things are not physical but are clearly defined. My remaining chapters deal with the other **must daily areas for me** that chapter one doesn't handle.

According to a 2007 Harvard Medical report "**strength training** is the most effective way to slow and possibly reverse the decline of muscle tissue, bone density and muscle power which dwindles over the years." Aside from disability which I associated with the weakened muscle discussion above is the fear of heart disease.

Heart disease is so wide spread that the slight mention of this word to me means I stick to a rigorous course of action to stave off the risk. The same 2007 Harvard Medical report on strength training spelled out more important information regarding the body's blood sugar. The report stated "strong muscles pluck oxygen and nutrients from the blood much more efficiently than weak ones. That means any activity requires less cardiac work and puts less strain on your heart. Strong muscles are better at sopping up sugar in the blood and helping the body stay sensitive to insulin (which helps cells remove sugar from the blood). In these ways, strong muscles can help keep blood sugar levels in check, which in turn helps prevent or control type 2 diabetes and is good for the heart. Strong muscles also enhance weight control."

When first diagnosed with m.s., the fear of disability planted a seed in my head. This seed continued pounding away at me that I might be sitting idle over a long period of time. This meant to me no exercise potential and heart attack city would rush in. In my early years with m.s. I didn't have a clue as to how blood pressure and cholesterol affected my heart and health. It was a common topic in the gym, on the streets, tracks and almost any public event. Now I have just a tiny bit of knowledge to recognize good numbers when I go to the doctor and gym. It is rewarding to visit my internist for my annual visits. Here I expect to receive consistent complimentary better than average scores for my improved blood pressure readings, cholesterol levels and overall conditioning. These annual visits were once required six month visits.

In my quest for consistently good heart rate, blood pressure and cholesterol numbers, I strive to keep a balance between strength training and cardio activities. Outside walking is preferred to inside walking because it gives my fitness and health goals a multiple effect. It also gives me a chance to get **exercise, sunshine and air**. According to Harvard Medical, sunshine assists in preventing many health problems. "It is a source of vitamin D."

Chief among Vitamin D's role is keeping bones healthy by increasing the intestinal absorption of calcium. At the same time that sunshine has been found to contain this positive news it has also been warned by experts that sunlight contains two forms of radiant energy. One form provides the energy your skin needs to make vitamin D but that energy can burn the skin and increase the cell damage that leads to cancer. Harvard further advises that to protect yourself, avoid the summer sunshine especially between 10 a.m and 2 p.m.

Harvard's advice further suggests to "wear a large-brimmed hat and a tightly woven dark-colored long sleeve shirt and long pants when you go out in the sun." There are other suggestions in its Health Watch reports.

Cleveland Clinic in a July, 2008 report focused on the protection of the skin from deadly cancers. It named melanoma in this report as the deadliest form of skin cancer. The report stated that "melanoma develops anywhere on your body but most often occurs in sun-exposed areas, such as the upper neck. Further, it warned that, melanoma attacks the skin's pigment cells and can invade the bloodstream, travel to nearby lymph nodes and then to the lungs, liver and other organs where it can be deadly." The report interestingly points out that the scalp and neck have a complex network of blood vessel and lymph tissue that makes it more difficult to detect and spread of melanoma.

Harvard's Health Watch newsletters have also reported that "Vitamin D may be good for a lot more than just the bones. Ample intake of vitamin D may help you fend off a wide range of conditions. These include colon cancer, diabetes and physical weakness in old age. Other studies showed that many people, especially as they grow older, have low levels of vitamin D in their blood. Our skin has an amazing ability to produce vitamin D when it is exposed to sunlight but with age, the skin becomes less productive. The problem is made worse by older people spending more time indoors."

My thirst for knowledge about bones expanded to the huge discussions about osteoporosis. Like so many men I initially thought of this as a "woman's disease." Reputable research has shown that it is more common in women than men and "it strikes women at an early age." According to Harvard Medical Watch, "the consequences can be serious and even deadly, ranging from height loss and back pain due to spinal fractures, to hip fractures that can lead to dependency and even death."

The warning from Harvard came as no surprise to me. My many falls in my earlier years with m.s. always scared me about bone fractures. It always amazed me that I got up quickly after a fall and at times noticed abrasions but never a long lasting soreness indicating bone fracture or other problems. More recently it occurred to me that my earlier and continued use of exercise as well as diet had influenced my resistance to health problems from these many falls.

Recently, I encountered a fall in a leading gym that scared the nearby trainers. A long extension cord in a dark area caused me to topple while going through a shortcut area in the gym to the next exercise routine. This shortcut was taken because of the crowded condition of the gym that particular night. This fall was a little bit different than previous falls because I received a large abrasion on my right knee. That required a trip to the nearby pharmacy for over the counter abrasion treatment and bandages. This treatment lasted the recommended pharmacist suggested seven days.

As usual my reading began. It was fairly obvious to me that something different had occurred this time but I needed that assurance this fall wasn't m.s related. After extensive reading and the quick healing process, I was comforted to learn it was not. More reading showed me that I had been spared a fracture because of my overall exercise and nutritional daily program.

Harvard Health Watch "stated that exercise and diet are ideal partners in efforts to enhance and prevent disease. What's good for your heart, circulation, metabolism and brain is also good for your bones." According to Harvard Health Watch, exercise increases bone mineral density. Harvard Health Watch further states that "bones improve with use like so many other parts of the body. In response to stress, they become stronger by increasing calcium." Most surprising to me was a comment from Harvard Health Watch in this same weekly newsletter "the reason why heavy people have a lower risk of osteoporosis than thin people, it's one of the very few advantages of obesity."

This Harvard Health Watch report reassured me that my weight-resistance exercise and walking were good combatants against osteoporosis.

Aerobic Exercises I Use To Keep Me Center Of My Target

Much needed exercise from **walking and biking** gives me **aerobic** activity aimed at keeping my heart and cholesterol in check and shape. Also, a plus is the lower blood pressure rate I maintain with the consistent walking and biking. A special 2009 Mayo report cited that "aerobic activity requires and utilizes oxygen. Regular aerobic exercise increases your aerobic capacity- or how well your body uses oxygen." "When your aerobic capacity is high, your heart, lungs and blood vessels efficiently transport and deliver large amounts of oxygen throughout your body."

Following my morning walk to get exercise, air and sunshine at least three days per week, I ride my **stationary bike** in my home gym. This bike ride has increased from a once low of six minutes per day to twenty minutes per day. Usually, these three days are my least heavy scheduled work days and at least one weekend day.

This bike riding has helped my walking and standing stability. Length of time and movement activity improves in both areas the more I ride. Flexibility of joints and ease of movement in my lower limbs receive noticeable attention by me and onlookers. Staggering and stumbling are nearly a thing of the past. Rarely, I encounter a stumble from an object in my path. Most of the times now I can avoid a fall from such an object in my path. This is the result of coordination improvement from exercising and **step exercises** which simulate **dance routines**. My goal now is to increase the dance routines since I recognize the positive effect.

The lasting effect of the exercising, walking and biking now holds my balance, coordination and stability three to four days. In the past, every other day and sometimes daily was a requirement. My quad muscles have received noticeable strength and mass visibility tests. Even my legs have begun to show improvement in appearance and strength.

My full conditioning program aims at levels that are acceptable to meet good health goals. I don't overdo it by pushing myself beyond unrealistic expectations for me and my health experts.

My medical professionals first began mandatory seeing me at six month intervals. Most now see me at one year intervals at their requests. Levels have moved steadily to become acceptable using a consistent approach for five years plus. This includes target heart rate, blood pressure rate, cholesterol levels, pulse rate and overall health.

Harvard Medical states that sound studies showed **aerobic** training is required to build optimal aerobic fitness. "Fit people are healthy people, with reduced risks of coronary artery disease, hypertension, stroke, diabetes, and mortality rate." Harvard's studies also show that is possible to get nearly all the health benefits of exercise without reaching high levels of **aerobic** fitness. Its reports even spell out that golf is "very beneficial as long as a player walks the course and plays two to three times per week."

The walking and biking activities are things I totally enjoy and can do regularly with very little deviation from my plans. These meet most of my **aerobic** activities. A recent American Diabetes report spelled out that these types of **aerobic** exercises (brisk walking and stationary biking) increase your heart rate, works your muscles, and raises your breathing rate. The report recommended a total of about 30 minutes a day, at least five days a week. Other significant **aerobic** exercises cited by the diabetes report are dancing, low impact aerobic classes, tennis, brisk walking on a treadmill, swimming or water aerobics.

Mayo Clinic in a 2009 report stated that "aerobic exercise includes some of the most popular and accessible activities you can do. It is important to your cardiovascular health and can help you lose weight, lower your blood pressure and decrease your risk of heart disease, stroke, diabetes and some cancers."

More **aerobic** activities included in my weekly plan are step and dance board routines using repetitions, and walking up and down steps. Plans are to expand areas such as dancing and include swimming in the not so distant future.

My core aerobic activities do not require the use of a gym. Walking outside is preferred to get the fresh breathing air. It eliminates that tight feeling of all body parts. It becomes a feeling of free flowing movement. Biking is done outside with the use of a plan old bicycle. On the other hand I mostly use the stationary bike the gym affords me at home and my away gym membership.

Strength Conditioning Exercises That Work For Me

Another major and valuable component of my total exercise program is my gym program. My overall gym program consists of strength conditioning exercises, flexibility exercises, aerobic exercises and balance exercises.

Scheduling flexibility plays a huge role in my daily lifestyle plan. At least three days per week are maintained for necessary core gym activities done in a fitness workout center. This center was necessary to get in much needed **strength training**. As defined by Mayo, "**strength training** involves the use of free weights, your body weight, resistance bands or weight resistance machine to increase muscle strength and endurance." Harvard Medical states "the health benefits of strength training (another name for muscle-building exercise) haven't been emphasized nearly enough."

Harvard further published that "strength training goes by several names: resistance training, progressive resistance training, weight training, muscle strengthening. The notion comes from the fact that your muscles are straining against an opposing force- gravity, for example, if you are lifting a weight." Harvard even cites some guidelines for muscle strengthening. Repetitions are "the number of times you repeat a movement." The groupings of these repetitions are called "sets" Its guidelines state that "as your muscles get stronger, you are supposed to choose the amount of weight that allows you to do only eight to 12 reps- and the last couple should be difficult. Two or three sets of each exercise are usually recommended." "As you get stronger, you are supposed to increase the challenge to your muscles by adding weight, because muscle needs time to recover, it is best to limit yourself to two to three workouts a week."

This concept of **strength training** was fully engaged and adopted by me when I used my friend as a personal trainer. This was done at the beginning stages of my rehab work over ten years ago. This trainer is still in the business and his program still works. Certain activities have been carefully added to the original program based on knowledge gained by me of what the various exercises do to my muscles and body. My trainer- friend established certain exercise standards for me. These remain in use today. Repetitions and sets are three sets of fifteen. The target for workouts are three per week. Every other day with a day in between workouts allows the muscles to recover, his terminology. The days in between workouts called "my days off" by him are normally used to do something aerobic at low impact. Again this was his initial recommended standard based on his work with collegiate and professional recovering athletes from injuries in more than one sport.

Choice of a gym initially for me was a major chore. Today's health and fitness society has expanded and made gyms plentiful and affordable. Two gym memberships are now at my fingertips nationwide at a monthly cost of what I used to waste in junk food and sodas weekly. Again, my exercise and nutritional lifestyle makes this possible.

Gym activities work best in the mornings for me. Sometimes, I have to shift these activities to the evening hours. The key is I get these gym activities in minimum three days per week. There is no compromise nor tradeoffs to ensure three days are attained. These activities are a critical part of my conditioning program and overall success of health and fitness plans. You can readily see from the strength training exercises that follow most of my conditioning is done on weight resistant training equipment.

- **Leg Press Machines** give me much needed leg strength on a regular and consistent basis. This machine was first began as a trial by me as an extra weight resistant machine after beginning working out on my own. When I saw and felt the initial effects of this type of machine I began using it every time I entered the gym. It helped when I visited other gyms with my female gym partner. Traveling I usually found that piece of equipment in the gyms used. This remains true today.

Over a five year period, this machine has taken away tingling in my legs. It has also provided the much needed stamina to help support my body mass while standing without swaying. Walking is readily made easier with more bounce in my step as I complete the exercise.

More in depth discussions with gym trainers and reading has shown me that leg press machines target the quad or hamstring muscles. This is the area that my sports medicine professional initially told me was my problem, a weak quad muscle. He was right on the money and used a series of manual strength tests to prove it. One of my doctors usually performs the same sort of tests.

The frequency of this exercise is no less than three sets of fifteen repetitions. Fun and ease of use makes this piece of equipment a mainstay. In my shopping, I readily look for a reasonably priced prototype of this piece of equipment for my home gym use.

- **Leg lifts** compliment the use of the leg press machine. This type equipment adds fuel to my quad areas. My old training buddy first started me on this piece of equipment in my pre-rehab years. This machine was literally hated by me. Hated mainly, because I couldn't even lift thirty to forty pounds on a single leg and sixty on a combo leg and weight machine my trainer wanted me to initially begin and stick with three days per week.

The leg lift machine became one of my most user friendly pieces of gym equipment over time. It is a mainstay in every gym I visit in and out of Atlanta. In my regular gym, I use two different types of leg lift machines, minimum three days per week. This machine comes in two basic models, a single leg with weights and combo leg with weights. The single leg lift for me targets 50 pounds per leg and the combo targets 110 pounds.

Repetitions used are three sets of fifteen for each type of machine and each leg. The only time I do less is I come in the gym tired. This is a rarity. Training and much heeded advice from fitness experts said stay away from the gym if you are tired. Use of the leg lift machines and reading the gym specs on the equipment taught me that they target the quad muscles. Most of the readers of my books and who meet me for the first time usually see me do a quad test with them. This test shows the improved strength and mass of my quads.

You would have to had known and seen me in my beginning stages of exercising to understand why I am so gratified to display this test. My illness (m.s.) had taken its toll on my quad muscles, particularly my left quad. The left muscle is usually in pretty good working order but it requires the fuel it gets from strength training minimum three days per week to function without a severe noticeable limp.

- **Leg Curls** are used to add fuel to my rear muscles in my quad areas. This exercise machine was my second most hated machine in the beginning stage of rehab. As time progressed the effects of the exercise was felt and visibly seen in my quad areas. This became a much sought after machine in each gym appearance. Today this remains true. It is still a tough exercise piece for me shown by me using maximum fifty pounds on each leg. The fifty pound increment was begun late 2008. Prior to this move upward, the poundage had remained at forty pounds per leg for almost two years. Repetitions are three sets of fifteen per leg. This type of machine is regarded as one of my required three days per week machines. The machine comes in two types. The traditional type called a bench leg curl machine is not as difficult to tackle for me as the seated version. It requires me to lie down face forward on a cushioned pad while lifting the weights with my legs. This was the only type available to me during my early exercise years until 2008.

Appearing in my gym spots in 2008 was the seated version. The seat makes it lazily enticing but it is a struggle for me to lift more than my 40 pound target. While struggling, I make this type of machine a mainstay each time I enter the gym and it is available for use. When both types of leg curl machines are available in the same gym I use both as part of my workout routine. The recommended standard of three sets of fifteen repetitions are used for both types of leg curl machines.

- **Calf Raise machines** target my calf muscles. This gives lift to my lower leg muscles adding balance and support for the upper muscles. Added to my strength training tools in 2008, I perform this exercise at least once per week. The machine is not in place at my regular gym but is available at a partnership gym. It is not a difficult to use machine and it makes the exercise fun to do. In a foot motion simulating walking , the front part of the foot (ball of the foot) near the toes meet a cushion pad thrusting it back and forth. This motion stimulates the calf area at low impact.

Three sets of fifteen repetitions with 90 pounds of resistant weight are utilized. Sometimes I repeat the sets since it is such a low impact type of exercise.

- **Abdominal machines** target my abdomen section. This machine does just what its names spells out. It works the abdomen section into shape. Observing the six pack guys and girls gave me every incentive to use this machine. At times my early gym days caught me peeping at some of these people to check out their routines and what made them successful. It quickly occurred to me that they were using similar techniques and consistency as I was. Three months into this type of equipment I felt a difference in my abdomen areas. Six months of working out in a steady and committed approach showed me huge gains in my abdomen area.

As you continue your gallant gym efforts, you usually meet someone of your kind, workout efforts, etc. This happened to me in my early stages of gym work after leaving my trainer. Actually I knew this person and I spent time with her prior to starting my gym habits. We regularly teased each other about going to the gym but we both took it to mean occasionally. Neither of us knew each other worked out so structured and military like. One day we challenged each other to a dual in her gym spot. Boy ,what a surprise to both of us. We were so encouraged by each other's performance that we decided to see my gym spot.

Readily, we saw the abdomen machine in my gym. We quickly decided and made a pact that no matter what gym spot we visited ,we would always workout on the abdomen machine every time we got in the gym's door. This has paid big dividends for both of us. It remains a goal today.

My regular gym spot now has two types of abdomen machines. One has a padded bar near the top of the chest in which the chin rests. This machine appears to pull the chest muscles into the workout. It is fun and so smooth ensuring that you lunge forward while resting on the bar. You get good abdomen action form this machine. The machine is a gym favorite of many gym workout artists, female and male. The second type of abdomen machine requires a little more effort and action. It requires the top body parts to dip forward toward the knees simulating sit up movement. Therefore, your abdomen area gets good action and workout. While using each of the two abdomen machines I maintain my standard three sets of fifteen repetitions. Oftentimes, I repeat the repetitions because of the ease of use of each machine. More importantly, the benefits and results I attain from using these machines are good reasons to do more reps.

- **Seated Dip Machine.** This exercise appears to get after my top back and shoulder muscles for added strength and stability of these areas.

My back is turned away from this machine while my arms and hands press the two bars down under weight resistant pressure. This is all done in a seated position on a padded bench. The position is not totally comfortable because the arm handles and bench thrust your neck and back forward. My weight increment used is comparably low to many of my other exercises. The weight increments chosen never exceed sixty five pounds. That is attributable to the fact that my back area is one of the stronger areas of my body. Given that knowledge from my trainer, I don't seek to build muscles in my back but to maintain my strength and balance in this area.

My shoulders are naturally stout (family male trait) but I seek to maintain good posture and strength by carefully going through this exercise minimum three days per week. Repetitions are three sets of fifteen.

- **Lateral arm raise machines** have been a part of my workout program since inception. My trainer introduced me to this type of machine at Georgia Tech's baseball training facility. It was a struggle during my initial six to eight months with him. However, I managed to tackle and enjoy this machine after meeting its challenge in my first YMCA training facility. Usually most of the gyms I frequent locally and while traveling have this piece of equipment as a mainstay. In a seated position both arms raise padded cushions under the weight resistant poundage of your choice. My choice is low fifty pounds and high sixty five pounds totally.

- **Pectoroid fly machines** target my chest muscles. I always wanted a pair of hard puffed out chest muscles. Never had I known the name of that area of the chest muscles until 2009. It just happened that I began working out on a neat looking piece of equipment frequented by several cut young ladies and guys. One day I decided to read the muscle visual area of the machine. This told me it targeted the chest area. One of my alternative gyms had this same piece of equipment and a second type. More reading and research added a new set of words to my gym vocabulary, pectoralis muscles. This major muscle section is defined as "a thick ,fan shaped muscle." It makes up the bulk of the chest muscles in the male and lies under the breast in the female.

Now, one of this type of the pectoralis fly machines is always a major part of my three days per week workout. Peaking out at 85 pounds maximum I work this weight resistant machine using both arms. It is a seated cushion machine which requires me to engage both arms on padded cushions using a swimmer's rowing motion. It is not a difficult machine and I have tested using higher poundage. However, using my trainer taught gym sense, I realize that more poundage is not needed. The 85 pounds gives me good resistant pressure without straining. My gym goal is not to seek building big bulging muscles. Instead I seek to remain firm and tone. Desired results are achieved using a self standard three sets of fifteen repetitions. Deviating from the three sets or reps has not been needed because I feel and see the results with each use of the machine.

- **Arm curls with free weights** are a core and constant part of my total gym program. Free weights and poundage were carefully chosen for me initially by my trainer. We began with various exercises using a low 10 pounds per hand and arm. These various exercises continue in use and the maximum poundage rose to a high 20 pounds per hand and arm with my trainer. Now I maintain 15 pounds comfortably with each arm curl exercise type. These exercises are all done in a standup position and function to provide lots of arm, shoulder and leg action.

First is the standard arm curl moving the arm forward from the chest and back with a fifteen pound weight in each hand. Repetitions are three sets of fifteen with no deviation. These curls have increased the mass of my upper arm muscles in a well proportioned style. Added to that has been noticeable upper arm muscle strength.

A second arm curl exercise uses forearm action. The movement is a hammer type action up and down. Again, three sets of fifteen repetitions get the job done. This type of exercise has provided much needed and increased forearm power using three sets of fifteen arm repetitions.

The third arm curl was devised to employ leg action as well as hands and arms. Using the right or left leg I move the leg forward while lunging forward with the free weight in each hand and arm. This exercise has given my trunk much needed strength and stamina while adding some aerobic impact action. Many gym trainer or on lookers have called this my boxer stance exercise. Three sets of fifteen repetitions are used for each arm and leg.

Final arm curl exercises consists of overhead action three sets of fifteen repetitions. Each arm uses the fifteen pound weights in an up and down fashion from the top of my shoulders to arm high. Consistent use of this type of exercise has gained shoulder strength and increased my lifting endurance. Prior to using this type of exercise over a period of time, I always grew weary of holding objects.

Flexibility Exercises for my Joints and Support Systems

Flexibility exercises usually begin my full gym workout routine. These types of exercises, called stretching , by most fitness gurus begin on a gym floor pad. Rarely, do I deviate from this fitness process during my three day minimum per week workout. In my early sessions with my trainer, I was fortunate enough to begin on professional style gym benches. It was a requirement to begin on the benches with warm towel treatments by him and his staff. These treatments relaxed my muscles and made them feel really loose and free when moving. Now, I enjoy this same freedom of joint and muscle movement without the warm towel treatments.

Using the floor pads today at home or gyms I engage in at least three variations of flexibility stretches using no machines. There are other stretch exercises that follow I use on some days to follow my mainstay weekly stretches.

- **Single Leg Raises.** While lying on my back I engage the use of a lifting motion from the floor toward my head. First , using my left leg in this manner , then the right leg in three sets of fifteen. The motions used simulate floor sit ups. Similar muscles are used including the abdomens. The big difference is the use of the leg muscles which is the primary focus of the exercises.

- **Side leg raises.** Swiftly I turn on the floor pads to a side position. Either left or right I lift my legs from the floor to the highest point my range of motion allows me in this position. Initially my range of motion allowed me to lift at a very low height. While consistently performing this exercise I have seen the height adjust itself to an improved position naturally.

▪ **Quad stretch.** On my all four pivotal points, I turn and begin a stretch using my trunk and quads. This is low impact activity but very good stretch action and creates quite a bit of stress action on the quads and knees. Over time, this action has reduced my stress action to a good comfort level in doing this exercise. While performing this exercise I usually count to fifteen for about three to five sets.

▪ **Step exercises** on a dance board received significant action during my workout days with my trainer. These exercise continued vigorously through my self rehab years. Now I have become slack with this exercise.

Three sets of plastic squares raise the dance board to a successfully challenging height for me. Starting with either the right or left leg, I begin the step exercise by stepping upward from floor to the board in quick and crisp action steps. Three sets of fifteen are my desired daily goal but I challenge myself to carry this exercise to my internal maximum. Many times this is more than the established daily goal. Coordination improvement, leg strength, and major balance improvement have been the result of this exercise. Internally, I know more can and should be done by me with this exercise. This is one of my major self-improvement goal changes staring me in the face.

My overall conditioning program keeps my body weight, body fat and muscle conditioning at ideal levels for me. My weight changes vary little, from one to three pound increments now when change occurs. During my battle years with m.s. around 2000, my weight kept changing up and down in five or more pound increments. Complaining to my mate became old fast. She firmly told me, "you are on medication and exercising. You must eat three square meals per day. Cereal is not a meal." The answer to her statements finally sunk in around 2004 when I began my full siege to get better.

The weight change stabilized with my changed diet and exercise habits. This included three square meals per day. Losing weight is not a problem for me. My struggle is to keep optimum weight and body structure. The Mayo Clinic published such a special report on achieving a healthy weight in 2007. This report included a chart with weight and height normality. Most internist medical doctors have the same sort of informational chart in their offices for viewing.

Exercise helps process my food into correct proportions for my body needs. It is a vital component of my daily maintenance. Measure of my success is critical. This is done with professional medical visits through cholesterol check, blood pressure, heart rate and other vital checks dictated by my medical professionals. When report of these checks vary negatively, it makes me that much more aggressive in my approach to do the things I must do daily.

A "lifelong exercise" approach has been credited to my exercise lifestyle.

CHAPTER 2
NUTRITION-LIFESTYLE CHANGE PHASES TWO AND THREE

In my early bout with multiple sclerosis, a successful nutritional lifestyle transformation resulted. It wasn't easy nor automatic to make this change. However, this nutritional lifestyle overhaul is the continuing result of my determination to stay disease free from multiple sclerosis and other degenerative diseases. This nutritional lifestyle change is a daily function. The change begins with the foods I eat (**lifestyle change two**) and extends to the juices I drink to my daily water intake (**lifestyle change three**).

Nutrition Lifestyle Change Phase Two- Foods I Eat

There is no compromise by deviating to other food or liquid choices. In a recent craze, researchers, writers and the health industry have begun characterizing foods into good health food choices and poor food health choices. So I will adopt those phrases for ease of reading this chapter of my book. Therefore, I mean by not compromising or deviating I don't satisfy my wants by giving in to poor food or liquid choices. Sticking to good food and liquid choices are optimum daily functions.

My daily food intake is usually done in three full meal increments: breakfast, lunch and dinner. My periodic function timetable to get these meals in is my most challenging daily chore. Most recommended periods are early am for breakfast, 11-2 lunch and 6-8 dinner. My timetable to get the morning walk and work schedule in limits me most Mondays through Fridays. Limiting means it puts me in a jockeying position to fill my time slots for these meals at normal time ranges. Through all the jockeying I make no compromises, that is, I get my three meals in. That means I sometimes exceed the normal recommended time periods.

What I eat and drink daily is most important to me. Early research on my part with m.s was challenging and I had limited proven research resources. This didn't deter me from reaching out to continue getting better and maintaining through proper nutritional methods. In my fourth year of research I reached the land of the giants in medical research. The names and written material of Harvard Medical School, Cleveland Clinic, and The Mayo Clinic became available to me. Many other names and written material became readily available to me but I adopted a consistent approach to receiving and reading the works of these three industry leaders over a two and one half year time period.

These research leaders usually portray their work in clear and concise manner, which makes it very useful for me. Needless to say I don't agree with everything I read nor adopt their approaches many times. My proven research and trials that worked for me to get better and live a better quality of life for five plus years have laid such a huge foundation for me. That it makes it difficult to alter my course at times. It doesn't mean I am against change but I ensure through more research that the changes I implement in my nutritional lifestyle have been well thought out and proven trial tested by the presenters. These nutritional lifestyle changes usually follow proven results and a close to natural lifestyle change.

Harvard Medical acknowledged in a special report entitled "Foods That Heal" there is a food- health connection. Harvard stated that "decades of research have produced study after study links between diet and serious illness." The special report goes on to highlight several health conditions that are most strongly influenced by your diet. It even gives a list of foods and nutrients that can decrease your risk of developing that disease as well as a list of foods or food components that increase your risk.

Cleveland Clinic published an interesting article in its May, 2009 Men's Health Advisor entitled "Eat Like The Greeks." The article suggests that the Mediterranean style of eating continues to show protective qualities against not only heart disease and cancer but also other maladies. Cleveland Clinic used a similar approach as Harvard to portray good food choices and what you can do. You will see a lot of natural nutrition in the Mediterranean diet. This same mode of thinking had been echoed in some of my other reading material.

It wasn't until late year five of my nutritional lifestyle change that I became familiar with the Rodale family name. This name had been right before me for years but I missed the opportunity to become more acquainted previously. This family's written material had assisted in laying the cornerstone to many of my lifestyle changes, particularly, exercise. However, I didn't connect the name until year five. Frequenting many magazine and book store counters prior to being diagnosed with m.s., I chose exercise magazines that talked about health foods you should eat while exercising. Similar to many exercise buffs I usually admired the pubs which showed the men/women with the interesting physiques. One publication that I regularly subscribed to for years was Men's Health.

During my early years with m.s., Men's Health wrote me and told me about a new publication they were introducing, Best Life. Immediately, I chose to subscribe to Best Life and remember even receiving its first issue published. Its contents and quality made it a good reading choice. Late 2008, I chose to research health oriented publishers in a nearby Barnes and Noble bookstore. This led to the Rodale name. Curious about the Rodale name I surfed the internet to learn that Rodale publishes, Women's Health, Men's Health, Best Life, Prevention magazine and many other household names. Immediately, I felt well connected to the Rodale Publishing name.

Best Life gave me many credible articles to read on nutrition. Usually, these articles became the focal point of many doctor visit discussions. One of the most dynamic articles I chose to archive appeared in its May, 2008 edition. This article dissected various good food choices into the type of body building immunity, enhancer and disease fighter types. Many of these were good food choices for me during my rehab years and even now.

In a more recent 2009 Healthy Eating Report, Harvard Medical stated "experts agree that the best way to get nutrients we need is through food. A balanced diet- one containing plenty of fruits, vegetables, and whole grains- offers a mix of vitamins, minerals, and other nutrients that collectively meet the body's needs" Harvard reported "it is not an issue of food quantity but food quality."

Breakfast is the catalyst meal for me daily. I usually cook this meal from scratch myself daily. This meal is so critical to my daily flow because of the nutrition gained and the energy it boosts. Rarely do I deviate from oatmeal as my fiber element each morning. This element is surrounded with fruits depending on the season of the year and availability. Baked wheat rolls are a constant. Grapes, bananas, and apples are usually in supply all year round in Atlanta. Usually, the red delicious apples are chosen because of the many benefits advertised. These benefits include inflammation fighting antioxidants, cancers such as prostate and swelling. That is why the phrase "an apple a day keeps the doctor away" was adopted, swelling. Other good sources of energy boosters and good nutrients for me are strawberries, peaches, plums, cantaloupe, melons, when available.

There are a ton of other good fruit choices that are promoted as good health choices. However, the above are my base. My occupation and self- employment has given me a definite advantage to eat breakfast in this manner. During my first three years I even had a range and surface unit in my office kitchen area. This alleviated the use of microwave. Today I usually bring the breakfast already cooked in a range oven or stove-top with me from nearby home when going straight to the office for work. My job requires me to take continuing education away from the office during certain times of the year. Again, Atlanta is equipped to handle most of my continuing education needs.

Occasionally I am lured away to a resort out of town for the same sort of educational requirements. Planning becomes my ally. Igloo chest containers have become a good tool for me to travel with because of their ability to maintain freshness and keep ice and hot or cold foods a long time. Also, I call in advance to determine the type of food served at the place visited and the preparation method. Certain food types such as grits have been occasionally substituted for oatmeal when traveling.

My do not eat list at breakfast meals is lengthy. No pork or beef products such as sausage, no dairy such as eggs, cheese milk or butter. Cereal is never eaten as a meal no matter what the advertising boasts. Care is exercised to avoid desserts of any kind even if displayed as a topping only.

Lunch is eaten daily as my largest meal. This mainstay has fit quite well for my energy and overall nutritional needs. Many days I get a normal time slot to do lunch. It is gratifying if I receive a visitor or client who comes in around lunch-time. That creates a window of opportunity for me to just stop all other activities including work and put all of my energy in getting a good nutritious lunch.

Most days, lunch consists of an all vegetable plate as my entrees. My usual favorites are collards, corn, green bean or black eye peas and sweet potatoes or yams. This is a four combination vegetable meal. In the absence of collards, I'll take turnips or cabbage or some other green leafy vegetable. Sometimes I'll do cabbage instead of beans or peas as part of my four combo meal. Corn bread is an entrée for me depending on the manner cooked. One of my favorite nearby lunch spots when I am in town working laughs because I always get two veggie egg rolls in addition to my four combo. Their workers now follow suit and I get the last laugh.

Limas, sliced tomatoes, broccoli, carrots are other nutritional favorites of mine for lunch. When there is ample lunch time for me (off work for lunch or some weekends), I cook my lunch ensuring it consists of a green leafy vegetable and some combination of at least three favorites (sweet potatoes, peas, green beans, sliced tomatoes, broccoli, carrots, lima beans). Eating in this manner is common place and a big part of nutrition one (food) lifestyle for me. Desserts have been absent from my lunch and other meals now for five plus years. Cravings for desserts are gone.

Maximum two days per week during wild fish season, I eat fish for lunch with vegetables and grains such as brown rice as my sides. Again my outside eating establishments for lunch are few and selective due to the ingredients they use in preparing the food. Tackling preparation of my own wild fish is fun. Such dishes as wild tuna, wild salmon, wild whiting have been prepared to a great degree of success. My cooking ingredients for these types of fish include, rosemary, thyme, parsley, lemon, garlic, onion, olive oil and 100 per cent juice as a base. Quite tasty.

    Traveling presents some difficulties at times but I usually topple these difficulties with pre planning and organization. The igloo container is my biggest ally for lunch and it never lets me down. Packaging neat veggie subs and 100% juices until I can get to a pit stop for replenishment if necessary is my typical approach. The usual travel pit stop for lunch is a vegetable plate consisting of my main favorites. Always, I seek the method cooked and ingredients used ensuring no animal fat.

    Dinner has become one of my favorite meals because it gives me options. By that I mean that breakfast and lunch have usually taken in most of the days nutrients required and demanded by my nutritional lifestyle change two. Therefore, little adjustment is needed to ensure that dinner contains a food loaded with missing nutrients. No, that doesn't mean that dinner is looked at as a cheat meal for me. It is just the opposite. Dinner is my lightest meal of the day in terms of the amount of food consumed. This means I can now eat a good food choice that is usually small in portion. My choices are not as rigid as breakfast with the required oatmeal, fruit and wheat rolls. The same can be said about lunch with the rigid requirements for vegetables.

    Dinner many times consists of a veggie sub or tuna sub sandwich with a side salad. This side salad sometimes is self prepared from fresh ingredients or picked up from the organic section of a grocer deli. The urge for baked or grilled fish is an option with vegetables or salad of my choice. Occasionally the option is an oriental dish of almond chicken or honey chicken, veggie spring rolls, broccoli and rice. Dinner can even consists of a large veggie salad and wheat based crackers. Sometimes, I enjoy a fruit or vegetable medley for a very good nutritious meal self prepared. Ahhh, look at the options and lack of rigidity.

The options even make traveling meals less of a hassle. Ease of finding most of my dinner items fresh at an out of town grocer or sometimes (restaurant) rests with dinner. Through it all good food choices and the will to stay disease free is utmost on my mind at dinner time, home or traveling.

Many times I have been faced with questions from readers of my book one on m.s., attendees of lectures or book signings. The idea to expand my thoughts on the foods and juices I eat and drink came about because of so many questions on my food and juice choices. This pole vaulted my thinking to present these foods and juices into a format that could readily be understood. Thus the choices of foods I eat and why I eat and drink them follow. The juice and liquid intake follows my narrative on my liquid intake in this chapter.

The next few pages highlight the good food choices in table format I have chosen. The tables include breakfast, lunch and dinner during the last two to five and one half years of rehabbing my body functions, building immunity and maintaining myself. You will also see in the tables why I chose each food and, that is, its health or fitness purpose according to my research. These choices were based on my last five and one half years of reading, research and personal consumption of the foods and nutrients in the tables.

The question of supplements comes to me each time I discuss my book or in casual food conversations. As a rule I have not done a majority of supplements in addition to my meals. A supplement chart is shown with the add-ons I have used with my meals. There have been no major attempts by me to use a large number of standalone vitamins or other supplements through years five and one half. However, continuing research has shown me to improve on good food and juice choices aimed at giving me proper levels of vitamins and minerals. Supplements such as barley, garlic, rosemary, thyme and a few others depicted in my chart have been in use since I began my rehab efforts over five years ago.

BREAKFAST CHOICES	
FOOD ITEM	**WHY I EAT THIS FOOD**
Oatmeal	Cholesterol control, heart health, colon health
Wheat Rolls	Fiber to calm inflamed tissues, colon
Grapes Dark red best variety	Eyes - cataracts, heart health
Banana	Source of potassium & for strong bones helps with nervous system and immune system
Apples, red delicious best	Prostate health, maintain reduction of all kinds of swelling
Strawberries	Vitamins
Peaches	Vitamins
Watermelons & honey dew melons	Bladder - water retention prevention and toxins rid kidneys of poisons
Cantaloupe	Helps prevent heart disease and stroke
Plums	Help keep bones strong and healthy
Cherries	Arthritic conditions, tendendinitis Topping for oatmeal
Raisins	Topping for oatmeal

LUNCH CHOICES	
FOOD ITEM	**WHY I EAT THIS FOOD**

Collards	Vitamins, Protein
Turnips	Vitamin content
Cabbage	Vitamin, bladder protection, infections
Corn boiled or cream style	Grain, colon, fiber, Inflamed tissues
Green Beans	Vitamin content
Lima Beans	Iron
Black Eyed Peas	Iron
Sweet Potatoes, Yams, Carrot Soufflé	Immune system health, cancer prevention
Sliced Tomatoes	Fight against degenerative diseases
Veggie Egg Rolls	Vitamin content
Broccoli	Strong bones, calcium content
Carrots	Cancer fighting credentials, eyes
Okra with tomato combination	Vitamin content
Grilled Salmon	Omega 3 Oil
Spinach	Muscle builder, bone density, prostate

DINNER CHOICES	
FOOD ITEM	**WHY I EAT THIS FOOD**
Grilled Salmon	Omega three content
Vegetable garden salad spinach, lettuce, tomatoes, carrots, cucumbers	Vitamins
Broiled corn or baked potato, baked potato chips	Grain, colon, fiber
Brown rice	Grain, colon, fiber
Oriental almond fried chicken	Heart, cholesterol, bladder, cancer fighting

Broccoli	Strong bones, calcium content
Sliced tomatoes	Fight against degenerative diseases
Veggie egg rolls	Vitamins
Vegetable medley: carrots, squash, tomatoes, cucumbers, sliced onions	Vitamins
Fruit medley: grapes, sliced apple, bananas, strawberries, cantaloupe, peach, plum	Vitamins
Tuna submarine sandwich with chips or broiled corn, or baked potato	Omega 3
Wheat based crackers	Fiber contents

JUICES	
JUICE TYPE	**THIS JUICE TARGETS**
Barley	Immune System maintenance
Apple carrot	Vitamins, iron, calcium
Green leafy vegetable	Vitamins, iron, calcium
Tomato Juice base	Vision, vitamins, cell maintenance
Carrot juice	Cancer fighting credentials
Berry juice smoothie including blueberries, strawberries, blackberries	Vitamins
Strawberry banana juice smoothie	Vitamins
Orange juice	Vitamins

SUPPLEMENT CHART	
SUPPLEMENT USED	**WHY I USE THIS SUPPLEMENT**
Parsley	Prostate health

Garlic	Arthritic conditions, blood pressure
Rosemary	Cataracts, memory
Thyme	Viruses and bacteria
Olive Oil	Bladder protection, cholesterol
Honey	Cataracts, germ fighting power
Barley	Immune system health
Almonds	Bladder and urinary functions

Harvard Medical's Men's Health Watch cited in a November, 2007 article that "the supplement industry is a $20 billion a year industry. Manufacturers and retailers assert many benefits and advertise these supplements aggressively. But is it good for your health? Are there other ways to gain benefits claimed for supplements is the question Harvard asks?" Harvard then turns around in this article and answers the question by stating that a good diet is a clear choice. Harvard cites Harvard's Men's Health Watch, July, 2006, as a reading source for more information. Regular exercise is cited as a good choice.

In an August, 2009, subscriber article, Harvard stated that it has "updated the reader comprehensive information on what vitamins and minerals you'll need, and details on getting the most benefit from your diet." "Good nutrition- and the way our bodies absorb and process nutrients- is a much bigger puzzle than simply getting enough vitamins and minerals."

Mayo Clinic in an August, 2009, Health letter did a feature on herbal supplements and risks to your health. The article stated that "the assumption that many people make that natural equals safe is not always the case." "Further herbal supplements contain ingredients that affect your body functions, much the same as prescription and non prescription drugs. When used properly, many herbal supplements may be safe and possibly beneficial to your health. However, a few can cause life threatening problems such as liver or kidney damage, uncontrolled bleeding, or heart arrhythmias." "In addition, some common herbs are known to seriously alter the effect of other drugs you may be taking, and can impact the safety of a surgical procedure." "The bottom line is that it is best to be open with your doctor in regards to your herbal supplement use, especially if you take medications and are about to have surgery."

Supplements used during my five and one half years target health through good choices. Similar to my core foods the supplements are researched for vitamin, mineral content and other health enhancement issues. Most regularly used supplements are used as additives and cooking ingredients. Olive oil is used to cook my vegetables and meats when I cook. Parsley, garlic, rosemary and thyme are used as cooking ingredients regularly. Parsley is even added to my breakfast oatmeal during the cooking process. There are other good supplement choices discovered during research. However, I haven't deviated much during my rehab, extended rehab and post rehab years.

Typical sample menus for each meal follows:

Breakfast

    Oatmeal with parsley (honey or raisins, or strawberries or cherries as topping)
    Honey wheat bread, no more than two rolls
    1 banana
    1 red apple
    1 cup strawberries 6-8 serving
    1 cup of grapes daily
    1 peach during season
    1 plum during season

Alternative breakfast meal

    Fruit smoothie such as strawberry, banana instead of oatmeal used about once every two weeks as a base meal instead of oatmeal other fruits –apples, banana, grapes always

Lunch

    Collards
    Yams or one whole sweet potato 0r carrot soufflé
    Corn (cream style or boiled)
    Sliced tomatoes (2-3slices)
    Green beans or black eye peas
    Veggie egg rolls (usually two)
    Corn bread

Alternative lunch meal

    Turnips or cabbage or spinach
    Cabbage
    Black eye peas
    Lima beans

Corn with okra tomato combination
Corn bread

Alternative lunch

Grilled salmon with squeeze of lemon juice
Brown rice
Veggie mix (carrots, cucumber, squash, broccoli)
Wheat rolls (no more than two)

Dinner

Tuna sub sandwich with lettuce, tomato, spinach, carrots
Side salad, baked potato or small bag potato chips

Alternative dinner

Oriental almond fried chicken
Broccoli, brown rice, 2 small veggie rolls

Alternative dinner

Veggie sub, baked potato

Alternative dinner

Veggie medley consisting of carrots, tomatoes, broccoli, spinach, squash, broiled corn, cucumbers, sliced onions

or

fruit medley consisting of grapes, 2 sliced apple, 1 banana, 3-4 strawberries, 2 slices cantaloupe, 2 slices peach, 1 plum

Alternative dinner

Grilled salmon, brown rice, side salad, lettuce tomatoes, carrots, cucumbers (eaten as early dinner meal only before 8:00 pm

Snacking is always a big issue when it comes to diets, health and food choices. It has always been a big issue for me because I always felt I would be overeating if I snacked. Therefore, my mindset and message sent to my brain is to rarely snack. It takes a major effort for me to remember to try snacking. It is not a daily function for me. At the most, I remember to snack twice per week. When I snack I stick with good food choices. Good snack choices for me include:

Fruits such as grapes, plums, peaches and watermelons during season

Nuts such as peanuts, almonds, pecans. Careful in my approach with nuts because of the heavy protein content, I have to fight off my thirst for eating too many of each. These nuts are some of my favorite good food choices

Wheat based crackers, chips with health oriented content

Old standby good snack choices include baked potato chips, popcorn and other cholesterol free products but mainly potato chips for my snack diet with little deviation.

Organic Choice

When confronted with the choice to buy organic, I usually buy in this manner. However, several factors come into my final decision including the producer of the product. Organic means the producer has attested to a certain criteria to grow and produce the food. Research is required to ensure that this party is certified organic. Therefore, price comes in to play because the parties have to command a higher price for their product.

The age old adage of common sense has to be employed in my final determination depending on the product. Interestingly about the time I wrote my own stance above about organic choices Cleveland Clinic wrote a late 2009 Men's Advisor. This Advisor contained an article on "Organic" "may not necessarily mean more healthful." "Cleveland Clinic's excerpt is cited from a report contained in the American Journal of Clinical nutrition. "The study authors research analysis found that foods produced organically are no more nutritious and provide no more health benefits than conventionally grown foods." There were more details and support about the findings in Cleveland's Advisor.

Nutrition Lifestyle Change Phase Three- Daily Liquid Intake

The daily liquid intake has been critical to my success to stay disease free and clear of flare ups from m.s. That is why I chose to classify this segment of my nutritional plan phase three of lifestyle change two, nutrition. This liquid intake includes water and 100% juices only. No other daily liquids have been used during my five and one half years of health and fitness plan. No sodas, alcohol content, coffee, just plain old 100% juices and water. This lifestyle change was first created to get well from m.s. symptoms suffered and experienced on a daily basis five and one half years ago.

High on my daily to do list is my daily intake of water. Water is a required daily must. My day is begun with one eight ounce glass of water before drinking any other liquid or eating any food. This process appears to get the body engine in motion like a well oiled machine. It gives me a gust of energy which propels me to read my daily scripture, then head for my early morning walk.

While walking I don't thirst quickly. Some mornings I end my walk with a ten to 15 minute stationary bike ride. By this time, I may sip another ¼ to ½ glass of bottled water. Usually I don't seek another bottle of (eight ounce glass of water) until I have eaten my breakfast.

Again, I stick with my old digestion techniques obtained from Dr. Lorraine Day. No water is drank until minimum one hour after eating and no more food until at least thirty (30) minutes after drinking. This agrees with my digestive processes greatly. Also, I don't experience pain nor the type of digestive problems I hear many people often complain about.

In a late 2009 UMM breakfast on the colon, I was reminded in my battle years with m.s. of the importance of the digestive system. It was very eye opening to hear from a talented Atlanta medical professional, Dr. Thurman, how large an organ the colon alone is. Its function is even more alarming. Now I better understand the liquid intake process because of the knowledge gained on the colon's function. For certain, the importance and necessity of my water and juice intake was reinforced.

Water not only gives me an energy boost but it assists greatly in my digestive processes. If I slack off on my daily liquid intake, my digestive system readily lets me know. Water is highly promoted by written and visible advertising for getting rid of body toxins. One gym I frequent two to three days per week has a special pre recorded message stating this throughout the day.

Cleveland Clinic in a June, 2009, monthly news Advisor warned that you can over hydrate. The article called drinking too much "water intoxication." It further stated "the amount of liquids you should drink depends on how much you sweat, the weather (hot, humid weather makes you sweat more, and the duration and type of exercise or activity you engage in." For me my water and juice intake peaks out about five maximum daily. Anything over five usually causes me to bubble up. Bubble up is my own term for "water intoxication."

Pure one hundred per cent juices are a perfect complement to my daily water intake. These juices are just as carefully chosen as my daily food intake. Juices have special purposes to assist body functions I discovered early in my rehab process and period. Therefore, my approach and maintenance plan has been to select a juice after reading the label and research its content purpose. Many times I have not only been amazed but steered into further research by finding the health connection of a particular juice content. Early on, my only purpose for buying a juice was to make sure it was antioxidant rich. Boy, was I surprised to find out that many 100 per cent juices do a lot more for the body.

A vivid example was the discovery of the contents of a green leafy vegetable juice I drank regularly for five and one half years. Among its contents are barley grass, spinach, wheat grass blue green algae, broccoli, garlic spirulina and many vitamins provided such as b6, b12, a and c. Cautiously, I am aware that all juices that say 100% juice do not provide all the good things promised for you. Some have high carbohydrate content or some other content displacing the content and intent of the juice potency.

Barley grass in a big way supports the immune system and wheat grass is a big help with m.s. symptoms. This fact has been supported by documented leading doctor discoveries and leading researchers' materials.

A chart follows with the juices I maintain as my daily use juices and what they target to help me with my overall nutritional program. Note that during my rehab period I sought to get in each of the juices listed daily. Today I have streamlined the number of juices and the amount of juices I drink daily. Bladder and kidney problems have to also be considered. That is where my urologist is most helpful in assisting me with the amounts and safe contents for my body specific.

Much research is done by me prior to using each juice. Today I have the resources of the big three research experts but my medical team is very reliable and resourceful. Juice contents really matters. It is always my number one priority to locate juices with 100% (percent) juice content from natural ingredients. Juice from concentrates is my least desirable juices. 100% juices help with the digestive processes and ridding the body of toxins daily. It is quite apparent that these 100% juices keep my body free of a lot of toxins.

Lack of colds, headaches, allergies and the normal seasonal and daily nuisances tell me much. It has been extremely comforting to me on a daily basis for five and one half years not to encounter these. No expert or doctor is needed to tell me I am on the right track when I have not encountered the above conditions for that long a period of time. However, I maintain my usual six to twelve months requested medical expert visits to ensure compliance and make sure some new undesirable isn't sneaking into the picture.

A better picture of my liquid intake can be seen in the following chart on daily liquid use.

CHART ON DAILY LIQUID USE

Water	One eight ounce glass before all meals, snacks and juices
Juice	One eight ounce glass fruit smoothie or apple carrot juice at least one hour after breakfast
Water	At least one half hour after juice and before lunch
Juice	At least one half hour after water and at least one hour after lunch
Water	One eight ounce glass late afternoon and at least one half hour after juice
Juice	Green leafy vegetable juice later afternoon at least one half hour after water and before dinner

Usually a minimum of five (eight) ounce glasses of juice and water are drank daily. I strive for six but top out at five most days.

Despite huge efforts to maintain myself at optimum performance and peak condition I have become aware of other medical necessity lookouts. Bacteria and virus infections come when you least expect them. My diet both food and liquid require a great deal of freshness day in and day out. My monitoring of where I buy my food and drink is critical. This requires the nosy neighbor approach. Many times I gain insight of a store or restaurant cleanliness from talking with neighbors or friends who shop at places. Sometimes I pick up information from frequent gym acquaintances who do the same sort of things. Cleanliness is not the only grading factor.

Factors such as grocer merchandising techniques must be considered. Rotation of products is important for grocers who sell fruits and vegetables. Many times you are able to spot freshness by appearance and decide whether to purchase or not. However, freshness can be hidden from the naked eye. Grade school taught me that germs and bacteria can't be detected by the naked eye. The vendor who sells the grocer or restaurant is equally important to me. Thanks to the internet and reading for knowledge I can acquire background on these sort of establishments after I become acquainted with their names.

My picky and peculiar nature sometimes causes me to throw out fruits or vegetables. This happens if I have the least suspicion of them not being fresh after I purchase them. Even the greatest efforts can't deter your body from setting up bacterial infections. My medical team taught me that in 2008- 2009. Juicing and water intake studies had to be considered for me to rid off recurring bladder infections. More than normal cautiousness and medical screening has been employed by me to stop or avoid a long-term problem.

Even CDC has been urged to keep a beefed up staff to watch for the many "new and old germ, bacteria and virus propelled hazards we face. This has to be implemented in my planning. That is, I can't afford to get sloppy or lazy on my planning nutritionally. After all I am no doctor and I certainly don't have the time and resources to do the 36 hours per day required to do a doctor's and researcher's work. My motive for maintaining myself and doing the laymen's research I do has come from doctors' written works such as Dr. Stuart Berger "How to be Your Own Nutritionist" and Dr. Joel Fuhrman "Eat To Live."

More than ever, I am totally convinced to get me a new power juicer and do my own juicing 100% of time. My efforts are in progress.

Weight Control

When I began my journey to seek a means to get better five and one half years ago, weight control and a desired weight was not one of my main goals. Vigorous exercising techniques had fully been employed by using the services of a professional trainer in my early bout with m.s. What was interesting then was that I did not know what I had, m.s. or whatever. As I journeyed on in my early years exercising, I saw favorable weight results, body mass and weight control. At times I noticed weight loss and my mate always urged me to eat three full meals. Friends and co-workers grew tired of me belly aching and told me to try snacking because I didn't eat enough. This was their judgment based on the fact that oftentimes I didn't eat all portions of my three meals.

Time and knowledge gained through reading and research showed me there was such a thing as a healthy weight. Mayo Clinic in a recent special newsletter stated "a healthy weight means you have the right amount of body fat in relation to your overall body mass." There is a body mass index that the medical profession and sports trainers rely on. Many doctors and sports facilities carry such an index in their offices. Even though this index is largely number oriented, this is an area I wouldn't dare venture into and strongly encourage readers to investigate with their medical providers.

Mayo Clinic further stated in this same report that "your chances of developing weight –related health problems increase as you get older. Overall, being overweight has many implications for your health and quality of life." Mayo cites that for these reasons, losing weight is a healthy goal for many. Mayo's reports continues to emphasize that health benefits such as increased self-confidence, energy, strength, activity and independence can't be achieved by "quick fix, miracle diets." Mayo cited "these sort of diets focus only on losing pounds. Most people who lose weight in this manner gain it back within a year."

Mayo puts strong emphasis on the same approach I began with and maintain in my overall success. "Lasting success in managing your weight involves a long term commitment to building healthy habits that last a life time." **"Healthy eating and physical activity- and staying motivated to continue these- are the building blocks of a healthy lifestyle."** Mayo drops a final bombshell in this report by saying "the intersection of all **three factors** is where you achieve a healthy weight."

Cleveland Clinic stated in a June, 2009 Advisor newsletter that "beverage choices play a key role in weight control." Cleveland Clinic's Advisor cited a new study reported by the American Journal of Clinical Nutrition. This featured the work of researchers who studied the weight and beverage consumption of some adults, ages 25-79, over an eighteen month period. The researchers found that sugar-sweetened beverages – soft drinks, fruit drinks, fruit punch or high-calorie beverages sweetened with sugar made a big difference percentage wise of calorie consumption. Significantly reported by the study authors were the findings that "reducing liquid calorie intake had a stronger effect on weight loss than did cutting solid calorie consumption."

My successful efforts to maintain myself nutritionally continue to be a tremendously useful guide for me five and one half years later. Most of my areas of health concerns are in check including weight control.

EverydayHealth.com reported in its October, 2009 edition on the question of How Does Diet Affect Your Multiple Sclerosis Risk?

"Doctors and other health-care professionals recommend a healthy diet to all their patients and especially to people with a chronic illness like multiple sclerosis. The purpose of such a recommendation is to promote a healthy lifestyle, rather than trying to prevent one specific disease. And in the case of multiple sclerosis, with the exception of including sufficient levels of vitamin D, not a lot of evidence is available to help understand how diet might play a role in the development of the disease."

The October issue alone presented the opportunity for someone with a medical background to write a book on m.s. Vitamin D appears as an imminent hope not only in this article but according to leading neurologist and internist whom I have recent spoken to. The article interestingly states "people with multiple sclerosis can benefit from keeping their levels of vitamin D high through their diet. Vitamin D is found naturally in certain foods (including fish, cheese, and eggs) and is artificially added to others (milk, breakfast cereals, orange juice, and margarine). But the easiest, cheapest- and possibly best-source of vitamin D is actually our own bodies: When the sunlight hits our skin, it triggers our bodies to make vitamin D."

Further this report sums up its recommendations as follows "the bottom line- until more is known about the effects of diet on multiple sclerosis, your best bet is to maintain a diet rich in fresh fruits and vegetables, lean protein, and whole grains and low in sugar and saturated fat. And boosting your levels of vitamin b12 and vitamin D through your diet and, in the case of vitamin D getting just 15 minutes of sun exposure a day won't hurt either (skip the sunscreen for the short period, though, as it blocks the rays that are needed for production of vitamin D)."

Well, EverydayHealth.com's October, 2009 report sums up many of my book one and two nutritional lifestyle goals. Someone is studying, listening and paying attention to the multiple sclerosis community.

CHAPTER 3
SLEEP'S ENORMOUS IMPACT ON LIVING AND FEELING HEALTHY

Comfortable with my sleep habits and patterns for five plus years now, I readily see the importance of good sleep and proper rest. It remains my mission to stay on a no less than six and one half hour per day natural sleep cycle. This cycle gives me refreshed energy physically and mentally to boost me into action for the next day.

Sleep Lifestyle

The next day's action plan usually determines my sleep planning mode. If my day is strictly a personal day, my mindset at bedtime is usually completely rest mode. As a result many times I wind up venturing off to sleep later in the night than usual. It is not uncommon on these nights that I don't see the bed site until well after my established norm of 10:30 to 11:00 p.m.

On the other end of the spectrum, a next business day requires a little more discipline for my sleep cycle and beginning go to bed sleep point. These days usually require myself getting into the bed no later than the 10:30 to 11:00 p.m. norm I have established for myself. Rarely is a wakeup call or alarm clock a must to ensure I get up timely. Furthermore, I usually feel the full effect of a good night's sleep. This full effect is no hangover, no sluggishness, no yawning for more immediate sleep. Yet, I have plenty of energy and alertness of mind to tackle the day ahead. My mood is good and eagerness to begin my daily activities is at hand.

My Immune System and M.S. Five Years Later

Sleep problems for me were rare prior to my diagnosis with m.s. During my battle years with the disease, sleep was affected using the medicine. The medicine would put me to sleep only to awaken sometimes, five to six hours later with major headaches. There were other times during the battle years when I awake with flu like symptoms. In addition I would be totally drenched with perspiration (night sweat). This drenching was so major that I would have to change night wear, shower and change the bed linen. This was frightening to my mate but we learned to cope.

Extensive reading and research on my own showed me that sleep problems could make my situation with m.s. worse. On the other hand, I was faced with a challenge to try a better sleep pattern and cycle. Ridding problems of m.s. conditions that I had experienced was constantly on my mind. Through my trial efforts and persistence, I successfully got rid of the sleep problems that m.s brought me in my battle years. Now, I am a "Gentle Ben" (BEAR) when it comes to sleeping.

My trial efforts and persistence did not come easy in my early years battling m.s. Early on I had to accept the recommendation of a true medical professional who had experienced traumatic problems with a degenerative disease. Even though this professional's disease (breast cancer) did not simulate m.s., it gave me a basis for finding answers and ways to fight the commonalties of my degenerative disease. In my soldier like approach, I proceeded to find the terrain (central nervous system) the disease lived on in my body. Starting at that point, reading began. This included reading every imaginable medical guide or book that I could find written on these subjects.

On this search and destroy mission, I found combatant sleep on the roadside. Initially I grudgingly placed myself on an earlier to bed approach, target times ranging from 9:30 to

10:30 p.m. Boy, was this tough at first especially pushing away from wind down things I had been used to such as television watching or exercising late with comrades in the gym. This required a total overhaul of my thinking and action plans for the next day.

After about three to four weeks of trying this earlier to bed approach, thirst for getting to bed early began to set in. My mate even began to adapt to the changes and made things easier. The earlier start for the day was tough enough at first. Early morning walking and gym activities began as eager tasks because everything I had researched and read said, must do. After the three to four week experience in doing things in this manner, it became a lifestyle change must.

One hard to get in change I made was going to sleep listening to soft music. This didn't go over well at all with my mate initially. She wanted to play various favorite artists of her own. My idea was to listen to mostly instrumental soft music such as smooth jazz. It took a while but this finally caught on successfully. The other way we wound up not getting much sleep.

Now, thirsting for sleep almost as much as I do water comes about when I get near my sleep cycle hours. Most times I don't make this time period before slumbering off. When I get home from a full day's work cycle or from a fun filled event or enchanting evening on the town, I look forward to wind down time. If wind down time consists of television viewing of a sporting event, most times I have to stay up for late night news to see who won the game. It could be super bowl, NBA playoffs, world series, etc. The outcome for me is usually the same, fall asleep somewhere in the middle of the game. Oh yes, there have been many times I had to find out who won the major sporting event the next day.

Using Interests and Hobbies to Round out Day Time Activities

Normally, I am not close to being a daytime sleep type of a person. My sleep cycle is nighttime driven. Using the daytime to catch up on lost nighttime hours of sleep can't be used by me. My daytime hours are filled with energetic and to do projects. These projects don't have to be work oriented. Finding fun things to do for me is easy. Fortunately, my interests are sparked by activities. These include participation, events frequented, or associations introduced by friends or mate. It is not uncommon for me to engage in a card or board game, read a good book or venture off shopping for clothes alone preferably. Many times this shopping alone turns into an uninvited twosome with my daughter or an uninvited threesome (her doing). Don't even mention going to see a youth sporting event, play or an opportunity to do volunteer work for youth or senior citizens. For those of you who wondered, I am back to playing golf and watching almost every sport imaginable on television or live.

Harvard Medical stated in a special report on "Improving Sleep" that "clearly getting enough sleep is just as important as other vital elements of good health, such as eating a healthy diet, getting regular exercise, and practicing good dental hygiene. In short, sleep is not a luxury but a basic component of a healthy lifestyle."

Harvard further states in this guide "Sleep decisions are a quality-of-life issue. Whatever your interests and goals, getting enough sleep puts you in a better position to enjoy and achieve them."

Bad Sleep or Sleep Deprivation

Insufficient sleep appears to be a center topic of almost every disease I research through leading medical journals or reports.

No doubt this has raised my awareness and thinking in my approaches to good health habits. It has led me to daily watch and improve my sleep habits. Harvard's guide shook me further when I read "new research suggests insufficient sleep increases the risk of diabetes, heart disease, obesity, and even premature death. Even a few nights of bad sleep can be detrimental."

Bad sleep to me means when I get up I feel sluggish, still want more sleep in a big way, or I can't function properly. Simple functions like walking may lead to a stumble, energy level says no go or my mental light bulb says cloudy conditions ahead for the day ahead. That is an absolute no go day for me without more sleep. It only took one of those days during my battle years with m.s. to heighten my sleep goals as tall as my exercise and nutritional goals. This has become a daily affair. That is, I maintain my persistence to get my daily six and one half hours plus sleep required for me to function adequately.

There are other concerns that leading researchers caution about sleep deprivation. Hand- eye coordination and reaction time studies linking sleep deprivation have been done. According to Harvard Medical, some significant studies have shown that driving abilities have been impaired by sleep severely. The studies showed the volunteers for the studies' lack of sleep had the same effect of drinking significant levels of alcohol. In other words, their driving abilities were so affected that "they could have been charged with driving intoxicated in most states."

Studies also have recently shown that "thousands of accidents are caused by sleep deprivation. A person's performance has been proven to be altered by lack of sleep. Such negative affects as mood changes and completing tasks requiring great detail have been linked to lack of sleep.

Harvard interestingly reported in one of its sleep guides that "partial sleep deprivation occurs when you get some sleep, but not 100% of what you need." This is referred to as "building up a sleep debt by experts." In this same series of reports Harvard cites sleep studies have linked "long term sleep deficits (s.d.) with significant health problems. Such health problems as obesity, heart health, mental health and mortality were listed as contributing cause recipients of s.d."

Age

Cleveland Clinic in a 2008 Men's Health Advisor stated that "age lifestyle habits also may alter your sleep patterns." Prior to her death, the songwriter, Aliah wrote a song that stays in my six changer, "Age Ain't Nothing but a Number." The meaning to most of her lyrics are very true. In my experiences with m.s before its attacks and after, I truly can say you must get proper sleep at every age level.

During childhood, medical and sleep experts say that newborns sleep off and on many times during the day. This disturbed sleep cycle changes with the infant's age in months. As the infant grows into its pre- school years the sleep cycle lengthens and naps set in at a shorter stage. By age six according to Harvard's sleep guide most children are awake all day and sleep for about ten hours a night.

Then comes adolescence. Reading says parents are still searching for answers as to why their teenagers usually need more sleep than they did as young children. Harvard says that adolescence is the most rapid period of body growth and development.

Adulthood usually brings on stability in sleep patterns according to the experts. Middle age years see nighttime awakenings as frequent and lasting longer according to Harvard. "It is common to wake after about three hours of sleep."

The later years of adulthood finds many people having difficulty falling asleep according to Harvard. Harvard's guide further says that "sleep experts agree that at any age, most adults need seven and a half to eight hours of sleep to function at their best."

Good Sleep - Better Habits

Good sleep comes with better sleep habits I found. Trial and error played the biggest role in my success. Simple things like cutting off all lights and moving my alarm clock so that I wasn't constantly peeping to see what time helped a bunch. Changing my time for my last water or juice to earlier in the evening helped equally as well. The soft soothing music is on most of the night while I enter sleep until I arise each a.m. It has a calming effect which gives me good restorative sleep. Most of the time I leave this music playing in the a.m. until fully dressed for work.

A big boost to my ability to calm myself down nightly and get ready for bed is the ability to clear my head. This is done by making all of the mental notes of the day left undone and putting them down on index cards for the next day. This written reminder clears my head and gets me ready for sleep mode at night. Rev. R.L. White made an interesting analogy in one of his 2009 telecasts. "Empty your head before going to bed. At the end of the day, he asks himself, did I do everything I could do today?"

Cleveland Clinic gave nine tips for better sleep in a June, 2008 Advisor:

- **GET SOME DAYLIGHT.** Open the blinds and enjoy outdoor activities such as gardening or walking.

- **LIMIT YOUR DAYTIME NAPPING** to no more than an hour or less.

- **AVOID BRIGHT LIGHTS AT NIGHT** especially after 7:00pm.

- **STOP VISUAL CONTACT** with things like computers, televisions, etc. at least two hours before bedtime.

- **NO SMOKING AND USING TOBACCO** products ever.

- **CAFFEINE** use should be limited or stopped. This includes coffee, soft drinks, etc. containing caffeine.

- **SLOW DOWN BEFORE BEDTIME** should begin within four hours of bedtime. This means stopping eating and exercise as well as other activities.

- **UNWIND BEFORE BEDTIME** including using your favorite relaxation technique.

- **GET THE CLOCK** out of sight to avoid the peeping for the time mentality.

One of my sleep habits still needs a lot of work, late night eating. Almost nightly, I eat my dinner meal later than 8:00 pm. This is primarily because I start the first meal of the day, breakfast so late. An early breakfast is a rarity unless I have an early am function to attend away from the office. The late night dinner usually does not cause me digestive nor sleep loss problems. Mentally, I know I am going against the expert recommendations. The types of foods I eat late nights play the biggest role in keeping me in a ready to bed mode. Dinner is my lightest meal of the day and the food types are carefully chosen.

The Boston Celtics professional basketball team reported in a 2009 televised game that they hired a sleep analyst in between the 2008-2009 and 2009-2010 seasons to study their players sleep needs. "Since they have a veteran team the sleep analyst said they required more sleep than previously required." As a result the coaches, trainers, etc. had begun requiring the players to sleep more after and in between games. They even passed on some in between team practices to allow them to sleep more. You might say the practices were being replaced with sleep.

The Celtics felt that strong about the analyst's findings to act in that manner. This significant move lets me know that sleep has been an important daily ally and must for me.

My research and daily adequacies has shown me that sleep requirements must be maintained no matter what age. Six and one half hours of daily sleep keeps me percolating at a very good pace with all of my activities and functions. When I get a good seven or more hours of restorative sleep, I feel unconditionally like a new person.

At least two to three days per week I strive to get between seven and seven and one half hours of daily sleep. Eight hours of daily sleep is the normal medical recommendation. Rarely, can I sleep eight hours straight through. Even elevated gym or outdoor activities don't propel me to require a solid eight hours. It is a nice thought but a rarity.

Observation and hind thoughts have shown me I usually get this eight hour sleep recommendation when I am on a holiday or work day break.

Making time to sleep has become an order from fitness and sleep experts. CNN fitness guru, Dr. Gupta T. warns workout artists to "make time to sleep and maintain the rest of your life."

Rest

At a crossroad one day in m.s. combat, sleep introduced me to his long time friend, rest. Their friendship became my friendship. After we saw so many commonalities between us we decided to stay bonded. Thanks to sleep I learned the difference between sleep and rest. Rest became a daily must. Almost instantaneously, I made a lifetime lifestyle commitment to get adequate portions of both daily.

Rest is achieved, mostly during the daytime hours for me. Time is made at least twice daily to stop work manually as well as mentally and sit idle. No work or to do list is usually on my mind during this process, just peaceful rest. The first rest time spot is mid morning. This is usually after I have attained a comfort level that my office workflow is in gear. Next I make sure those gears are steered toward the right track to achieve the day's goals.

A larger portion of rest time is allocated to the afternoon when the day's workflow has simmered down. This is usually after one of my clerical staff members has left for the day. This period is dedicated to listening to smooth music of various kinds. Many times I dedicate this period to watching comedy on television or dvd. At least thirty minutes to one hour per day is my target. Many days I reach this target.

However, a pleasant obstacle has cut into my afternoon rest time period as of late. My daughter and I work the evening shift together by choice. Therefore, I have to make myself available to her for question answering and training techniques. Don't get me wrong, I am one of the happiest dads in the world right now. God has blessed me with a daughter who did her undergraduate work in Chemistry pursuing a pharmacy career. After a few years of working for major metro and national pharmacy chains she became a certified pharmacy tech.

Later, she got her master's degree in Business Administration. This masters in Business Administration was a planned step by her in setting her goals to succeed her dad in our 100% family owned Tax Accounting business. This took no coercing and asking on my part for her to enter the business. She made this decision on her own. When she presented her wishes and demands to me over six months prior to coming to work, I thought I was listening to the reincarnation of some of my ancestors.

Her level and pace of learning the work and business has yielded good results for the business and me. This allows me to enjoy a bunch of music or television/dvd watching. All is done while she is working on her own. At the pace she is going, much rest is assured ahead for me. What a blessing!!!!

Relaxation

Long time pals sleep and rest spent an enormous amount of time with me during my m.s. rehab years. Their friendship remains eminent in my life today. Such an extensive engagement taught them a few things about me. They knew through their experiences about the successful work of their combat buddy, relaxation.

One day in late 2008 they introduced me to relaxation. This actually became a reintroduction we all found out later. Meeting relaxation this time took on a whole new meaning for me. It meant expanding rest into a different level. That is, I stopped forcing myself to stop each day and sit idle. It became a natural practice to take time for myself to add fun things I enjoy participating in to my rest period.

These fun things lift my spirits and motivate me to look forward for opportunities to add relaxation periods in the coming days ahead. Music is a natural for me. Many clients have been amazed and in awe of my music collections of more than one flavor. This craze for music grew with age and association with musically oriented frats, friends and clients. Listening to music or grooving to the lyrics completely refreshes me mentally. It is no challenge and effort to get into the flow of music for me.

Some days I lull into a comedy state. When this happens I pop in one of my collection dvds so that I can laugh. Many times I find myself laughing so hard at simple things that comedians make funny. Laughing releases me and launches me into a state that I forget about the past days concerns and cares.

On non workdays, I become a participatory relaxation partner. That is, I seek something I can do physically or mentally that creates a fun to do project for me with my mate or alone. These funs things appear naturally according to mood and the pace of the day. Most days it becomes a leisurely stroll through a picturesque site of greenery, color, park or neat one time previously seen site. At one time this sort of stroll was a struggle just to move one foot in front of the other.

Today the stroll is comfortable and at a leisurely pace. It is activities like these that not only reinforce you mentally and physically. They also show you that you are with the right person in your life because of their patience with you. This patience persists even if you can't compete step for step with them. Mutual patience desiring to spend time with each other through all trials and tribulations creates a bond beyond measure.

Sometimes I am pointed to go visit a not so frequent gym spot. It may be to do some simple stretch exercises with my mate or watch some of the new dance practice routines. This keeps the luster in the relationship and sparks new ideas. On other days it is a visit to a mall or a new shopping spot just to see what's new. In metro Atlanta, we are fortunate for new sites to appear from one visit to an area of town until your next visit. So this becomes a fantasy affair many times.

Sprawling Atlanta presents such unique opportunities as collegiate or professional sporting events on many levels. Don't even mention AAU, Olympic qualifying, youth and high school sports of many proportions. Relaxation at the event of my choice is at hand year round.

New opportunities keep arising in my quest to get relaxation. Opportunities such as revisiting playing or viewing golf are at hand. That is where relaxation and I first met, at a middle Georgia golf resort community years ago. My job position in those earlier days with relaxation required extensive travel throughout six southern states. Relaxation was no doubt stationed at a major army facility less than thirty five miles away. The golf community was a regular refuel stop for relaxation and myself.

We both managed to pick up and maintain quite a few clients and relationships at that refuel stop. It was a good fit and friendship then. Today it is a requirement that we maintain and nurture this friendship on a long term and lifetime basis.

CHAPTER 4
YOUR OWN STRESS-LESS-NESS GAME PLAN

Having accepted my diagnosis with m.s., it became quite apparent to me that I could live with m.s. a sustained time period. On the same plane, stress had to go for life to continue. The question now and then is how do you manage stress and live a quality life?

Stress Test Game Plan

My team of medical experts who diagnosed me with m.s. could not give me a strategy nor plan to handle stress. They managed to tell me stress was known to be a contributing cause to what I had, multiple sclerosis (m.s.). They admitted no real medical cause or cure for m.s. was known. What was even more disheartening was they could not even give me a referral. So I sought the services of proven experts in their fields eager to take the challenge of establishing a stress management game plan.

Exercise was the unanimous choice for ring leader and general of my stress management team. Primarily chosen because of its aggressive nature and first successful m.s. assaults early in my life, exercise stood out. Exercise developed its own way of reaching team members, air and sunshine. Together, they helped me immediately name the game plan stress-less-ness.

Carefully chosen and deployed into action were nutrition gems proper foods, water and 100% juice. Sleep had its own team of experts, rest and relaxation. The right attitude and faith were naturals since they seem to come from within.

These internal driving forces no doubt pull together your team and give you that winning desire and competitive edge. This dynamic team is a formidable force in place in my daily lifestyle today.

"Stress Tickers"

Re-examination of myself, personally setting goals and gauging progress is just a part of my competitive nature. Constantly, I look at personal life achievements, work habits, work environment, work goals and achievements to determine if they are satisfactory to me. This evaluation is done with a great deal of thought. Sometimes, notes are made on key concerns I feel better progress or more work on my end is needed. In those situations I may follow up with outside assistance. Documenting everything is not always the case because you can overdose yourself. This causes boredom, a stress ticker.

My definition of stress ticker is something that signals stress is ahead of what you are doing or facing. Harvard Medical's recent Stress Management Guide gave an interesting definition of stress as "an automatic physical response to any stimulus that requires you to adjust to change." When you examine my stress ticker definition and Harvard's professional stress definition you can create your long list of stress causes.

My list includes: unpaid bills and no money, poor relationship, traffic jam, work deadline closing in, too many people demanding my time now, IRS wants money I don't have, discovery of a serious illness, and so on. Through it all, you must learn to adapt to this change/request or get eaten alive. When confronted with these sort of challenges, I create a plan of attack. Most of the times, I wind up breaking the problems down into manageable parts, not swallowing the whole. This is the same as the old school, backing off or regrouping.

M.S. in my life causes me to stick to my daily plan to avoid stressing. It is less of a chore that way. Such a lifestyle gets the word chore out of the process. My lifestyle includes exercise on a daily basis. It would cause stress if I could not exercise on a regular basis. This lifestyle change has been in place ten plus years. Exercise has not only retooled, rehabbed and reshaped my physical side but it has a done a mental job as well. Mentally, I get refreshment from the effects of regularly exercising. At least three days per week I engage in strength training in a gym. This core part of my fitness routine shapes me mentally. It is a reward I look forward to before and after each training session.

A reward of knowing I attain something each time I visit the gym without coercion from anyone is gratifying. Comfort and peace within comes with knowing I am doing something to keep myself replenished and refurbished. The reward of good health and physical well being are ultimate rewards. No m.s. challenge has visited me in five plus years attributable largely to my exercise and fitness lifestyle. These rewards alone deflate stress for me.

Along with regular gym exercise, I strive to walk daily. Less than twenty days per year I do not walk outdoors. This walk is somewhat brisk now and not tentative. The air I get outdoors helps retool my energy level and air passageways internally. On days I get sunshine I am able to get vitamin D. Recent studies and research shows that this is good for m.s. and the body's bone structure. The reward I get from walking is knowing that at one time I was scooter ready and never envisioned being able to walk again. Nearly five successive years now without any assistance I have walked. The walk is not always as steady and swift as it once was but I am able to walk.

My nutritional team keeps me in full gear and well balanced. My good food choices nourishes my body and no doubt keeps me disease and stress free. By eating the right foods I attain a comfort level mentally that I am doing well because of these nutritional habits. This mental comfort level expands my thinking and reassures me no major disease or setback has visited me in five plus years. Extra efforts are made daily to maintain these good food habits as a result.

An even bigger challenge presents itself daily to consume the needed water and 100 % juice. These nutrition assistants not only add fuel power but helps rid the body of daily toxins. My timetable between juicing, water and food intake leaves me very little time to be hungry. There is no rush to eat or drink. A good steady level of these nutrients keep me from stressing about food intake and wondering am I doing the right thing.

Then comes the daily bout, maintaining a happy medium of work and play. Often criticized for my long hours of work habits I quickly learned to adapt and change in my rehab years. Today I lead a much healthier lifestyle because of these changes. Work lifestyle changes created better organization and implementation of better planning techniques. The long work hours are a rarity and I utilize technology to give me an added advantage.

The once used super early in the morning technique is gone. This was employed at the beginning stages of acquiring and implementing get well methods.

Working now more productive and efficiently gives me a more satisfied feeling of my overhauled work habits and daily efforts. Performing the work accurately and in big amounts was never the problem. However, it took discovering some techniques that gave me more time for myself gradually. This has become so satisfying that I refuse to give it up. Now, more time is allocated to planning and strategizing to find ways of improving good to better.

It was a wrestle to the finish line with stress in my early rehab days. This wrestle gave me the vision to start unusually early to get my work done in a stress free environment. Today, I am better equipped to mentally start early on my projects requiring more attention to detail. This early start is usually my normal wake up time. It is no struggle to get exercise and walking in on most of these types of work days. However, if I sense a slight feeling of being pushed or stressed to get my workout and work done, I regroup. It becomes a simple matter of going forward with the work and delaying the workout to an evening time slot but not too late.

Many times this early work start is begun at my home office giving me an added advantage of no distractions nor stress tickers. Usually, I am successful to get these sort of projects done in less than one half the time it would take in a high traffic environment. Allocating the proper time to my work assignments, special projects are common. This giving enough time process has become a part of just about everything I do, work and play. Leaving early for appointments, personal (doctor, dental appointments, sporting event, church) or business (visit a client, business lunch), receive the same sort of commitment.

The hurry up and get ready approach is taken out of the process. Further, this allows for a mistake I make along the way in locating a not so familiar location or a wrong turn. Further it could be an unexpected traffic delay or police identity check point. Either way I am usually covered leaving early.

Even though my work habit overhaul began in 2004, some helpful things happened as a result of some unrelated plans. Carefully planning an office move with my daughter in late 2006, early 2007 we finalized the office move immediately at the end of tax season. This move proliferated the work habit and environment overhaul. By that I mean this move took away some of the things the old workplace had that lured me stay longer on many days.

You must first understand the old work location was a standalone house occupied by my business only. This gave me a comfort level to go and come as I pleased. Coming was easy but going was usually the problem. Usually, I maintain a television, cable ready and music component equipped. What a problem on most workdays. After work hours some neighboring clients felt I was working long hours. No, I was usually engaged in television watching or listening to music. Sometimes I even had visitors assisting with the problem, that is, enjoying the same amenities. Some even came to tell me what time the next movie or game was coming on.

The old location had an oven and range fully operational. Oh, yes, I even added a refrigerator and had two once my daughter graduated from college. Matters were made worse by the fact that one of my sofas was actually a sleeper sofa, heavier and more sturdier than any other asset in the building. You already know about my sleep habits thanks to the efforts of my friends in Chapter three.

The new location is extremely comfortable but is in an office park. My space is completely private, quiet and convenient. Much of the home atmosphere taken away by the move keeps me in a go home after work mode. The television and music are still in the office but I look forward to going home more and earlier now to enjoy these sort of activities. The office atmosphere helps with that, you are through now, don't you have a home to go to ? In other words, leave, I see you early in the morning and all day long.

However, my biggest obstacle now is beating sleep and friends, rest and relaxation out of the new office door. This is the case to go home or to one of my spots away from work. It has come to my full attention more rewards are attained at home doing these things. Added benefits usually come by going home to rest and relax. This added leisure time is a great reward to myself. During this leisure time I find many simple fun things to do that never entered my mind prior to my new leisure time opportunities.

Enjoying doing nothing sometimes is so gratifying. Just come home with nothing purposeful in mind to do. No television, no music, nothing but the sound of nothing and yourself. Before that gets old, that is, no consecutive daily nothings take place, I quickly turn to something to do different for leisure each day. It is usually a non thought process, just whatever I choose to do on a given day. It can be listening to some of my favorite music artists on a different day. On a different day it can be engaging in television watching, mostly humor or sports related programs.

Many times, I find myself turning away from a sporting event including one of my favorite teams. As I told my banker and daughter, it becomes stressful watching your favorite team of any sport falling behind or barely in the lead. Nail biting, jumping up and down and sometimes angrily throwing things at your television set or wall are not my ideas of leisure or relaxation.

Calmly, I engage in leisure activities that keep me toned down. This approach sometimes leads me to do something creative. Trying a new dance step becomes interesting in moments like this particularly if no one is around to judge your stepping ability. A green thumb is a part of me. So my mood sometimes leads me to the local gardening store depending on the season of the year. That takes quite a bit of planning but it is a rewarding experience to nurture your plants and watch them grow.

There are moments that I find myself in the kitchen trying out a dish my mate said I couldn't handle. There is also the challenge to myself on doing a different dish than the normal. It is not uncommon that I find myself writing for leisure. Expressing myself in words and getting the thoughts out of my head sometimes refreshes me mentally. This is not an everyday nor every week occurrence. Writing is a mood affair but you better take advantage of that moment when the mood hits you for full effect.

Sleep's friends rest and relaxation keep me occupied a lot these days. Both have these sneaky and enticing ways of grabbing my attention in the middle of a big project. You hear these voices inside your head calling you and reminding you of the fun ahead after finishing a project. Most of the time, this puts you in a position to take breaks and use some relaxation techniques. Sometimes, it is simply a matter of putting on a smooth favorite music cd to work by or better stop and just listen a while.

For sure their gallant efforts continue to show me their collective efforts have kept me disease free five and one half years plus. Harvard medical placed a long list of medical conditions linked to stress in one of its recent stress guides. This list included such health problems as-

ALLERGIC SKIN REACTIONS
ANXIETY
ARTHRITIS
CONSTIPATION
COUGH
DEPRESSION

DIABETES

DIZZINESS

HEADACHES

HEART PROBLEMS such as angina, heart attack, and cardiac arrhythmia

HEARTBURN

INFECTIOUS DISEASES such as herpes or colds

INFERTILITY

INSOMIA

IRRITABLE BOWEL SYNDROME

MENOPAUSAL SYMPTOMS such as hot flashes

MORNING SICKNESS (nausea and vomiting of pregnancy)

NERVOUSNESS

PAIN OF ANY SORT (including backaches, headaches, abdominal pain, muscle pain, joint aches, and some others)

POSTOPERATIVE SWELLING

PREMMENSTRUAL SYNDROME

SIDE EFFECTS OF AIDS

SIDE EFFECTS OF CANCER AND CANCER TREATMENTS

SLOW WOUND HEALING

TROUBLE SLEEPING AND RESULTING FATIGUE

ULCERS

Even though multiple sclerosis is not on this long list, all leading research guides implies stress' connection to m.s.

Harvard does say in this same guide that "studies show the immune system is affected by both short term and long term sources of stress. The ability of the body to resist disease remains uncertain."

Who would want any of this long list on their starting five, starting eleven front or any set front to fight or defend. This is why I choose to stay with my daily top ten combatants carefully analyzed in the seven chapters of this book.

Harvard Medical exhibits tireless warning efforts of the disabling and silent killing effects of stress. These efforts are also seen in a special stress relief section of its stress guide. The guide lists "ten common stressors" and gives suggestions to assist with each. The ten are:

FREQUENTLY LATE

OFTEN ANGRY OR IRRITATED

UNSURE OF YOUR ABILITY TO DO SOMETHING

OVEREXTENDED

NOT ENOUGH TIME TO STRESS RELIEF

FEELING UNBEARABLY TENSE

FREQUENTLY FEEL PESSIMISTIC

UPSET BY CONFLICT WITH OTHERS

WORN- OUT OR BURNED- OUT

FEELING LONELY

Harvard's special relief guide also points out some more valuable stress fighting techniques that could assist with stress. These key areas listed in its stress guide are: "meditation on the go, mini relaxation techniques, keeping a gratitude journal, deflate cognitive distortions and make a worry box."

The single most interesting point to me in Harvard's Stress Management Guide was the topic on the "Power of Prayer." When I first saw this topic I said to myself, now, this big mecca and conglomerate of knowledge is going to give me an intellectual lecture on prayer. After reading this section I quickly regained my focus on why I chose Harvard as one of my top three research experts to rely on in furthering my research and writing efforts. Harvard quotes in this section "several large studies suggest that people with an active religious life stay healthier, live longer, and be happier." Comforted by this phrase alone, I moved on.

Oftentimes, you can find yourself flooded with choosing from the various smor-gas-boards available to remedy stress. Outside assistance is a matter of personal choice. Busy and chaotic environments create imbalances in our daily lives. Decisions must be made on how to deal with these imbalances or get swallowed up. The songwriter gave me a personal remedy when she wrote the lyrics "THE GREATEST LOVE OF ALL IS LEARNING TO LOVE YOURSELF."

This love for myself follows me in all of my endeavors. It leaps to me in learning to nurture myself in stressful situations and conditions. It follows me in my career, relationships, social activities, leisure activities and spiritual life. Included in this long list should also be thinking time for myself, relaxation exercises and creativity time.

Adjustment and change are remedies for me in dealing with stress tickers. If it is work where I see stress building I seek to restore divine order to the workplace immediately. Calming myself, I stay attuned to my feelings and emotions despite the weight of activities. An anxious decision is seldom made because it is usually a wrong and costly one. Fear and turbulence are not my comrades. Therefore, I usually proceed in peace to arrive at harmony.

Keeping the glue to a relationship is a massive stress ticker I have to deal with daily. This challenge many times has led me to regroup to my own plans. At times it has been a cliffhanger to a relationship. Careful thought and consideration prior to a final decision is always given by me. Early decisions and no pondering around has led me to many good decisions in relationships. When it is something I am against doing, I throttle back. That, I withdraw myself from going forward with it by discretely letting the other party know I have other plans. This is usually tough particularly when it is a friend. A mate dictates a different plan and route altogether. There is usually a compromise that we both agree on that suits us better in the long run.

An interesting analogy was given by Rev. K. Lee on local Atlanta television in 2009. Rev. Lee stated that "it is easy to develop relationships with people who are:

1. **skeptical of you.** That is, they don't trust you. An example is the limp hand shake you receive from people you meet the first time or weak hug.

2. **people who are experimental or who put conditions** on a relationship. An example is a person who tells you he or she is so in love with you but uses a conditional phrase which usually begins with but. This conditions means the relationship will work as long as you continue doing a certain thing for the other party.

3. Rev. Lee's third easily made type of relationship is people who are **sacrificial** with you. He used Daniel and his three Hebrew friends in dealing with the King's guards. They asked the guard to deny them The Royal

King's food and give them food and water for ten days instead."

A rock solid principle I have is not allowing myself to get sucked up by stress. "You put pressure on yourself in most situations has always been expressed by generations of my family." You have to stick to your guns or own decisions often times when opposed in relationships- family, friends, mate or work. Always make sure your decision has good merit and makes good sense is my firm belief. If it is work related, this basis may require some additional proof support.

Faith in yourself and decisions are vital keys to your own foundation. This foundation borders stress and me. Home is my palace and place I retreat daily to seek peace and relaxation. My home affords me the opportunity to rest my body, mind, and rekindle my spirit on a daily basis. This further allows me to release my cares of the day and reenergize my thoughts. Stress can't operate at home or I will have to move first. This firm rule boldly keeps stress away from my door.

CHAPTER 5
THE RIGHT PERSPECTIVE-ATTITUDE

In a UMM breakfast setting, 2008, Dr. Cooper pointed out to the group that you should develop a "state of mind approach" in goal setting. This "state of mind" approach should be used to launch a healthy lifestyle he further roared on. "Attitude is critical in this process he injected."

Attitude is the glue that bonds my daily healthy lifestyle. This attitude defines the way you think, walk, treat your fellow man, maintain your relationships and maintain yourself. Adopting this sort of lifestyle is a personal choice. Attitude can easily be persuaded by social influence or experiences. However, consistency is one of the vital components that keeps my attitude in check.

Equally challenged daily to get off track on my goals an attitude lifestyle usually forbids such moves. These daily goals include health lifestyle, spiritual lifestyle, mental and physical preparation, fun, relaxation, occupational and reaching out to others. It is a huge reward to attain these goals daily. The measure of my success is reaching these heights daily.

Each day I get up early with my things to do already engraved on my forehead and on my chest (a figure of speech only). First priority is get that first eight ounce glass of water. Next it is get to the daily scripture reading in one or two of my little biblical arsenals. Next, out the door I go to the track to do my three fourth to one mile daily walk.

Failure appears to set in if I don't accomplish the above first each morning. Alternative planning is made for not accomplishing walking. Usually, plans are made to get this in after a work day. Most times when the morning walk is missed and alternative planning used, it doesn't happen. When the walk is missed I feel like I have failed myself and missed an important daily health piece.

Attitude remains a constant in all of my daily approaches from my morning hike to ending my work session in the evening. Needless to say you want to maintain a positive attitude but you have to realize that your day and best efforts are going to get turned around some days. When this happens alternative planning must come into play. Some call it making changes or contingencies. In sports, it is called having reserves in place to replace the injured, tired or plain old not getting the job done change.

Alternative planning for me consists of having a different time or day planned in case I can't stick to my regularly planned schedule. Examples can be seen by looking at my liquid intake, exercise, sleeping habits and spiritual nourishment.

Liquid intake optimum for me is to get that first glass of water in before leaving the inside of the house. A few days I miss this important first glass of water. When this happens I adjust the full day's liquid intake. No less than three eight ounce glasses of water and three eight ounce glasses of juices are drank each day. There are some days I get one to two glasses of additional water and one to two more glasses of juice.

In my liquid cycle, I never drink liquids and eat at the same time. It is my practicing eating and drinking habits to stick to a norm developed during my rehab years. That is, I drink liquids minimum no less than thirty minutes before I eat and no less than one hour after eating. This practice continues throughout a twenty four hour cycle, 24/7. It worked to get me well and avoid other side effects that could have resulted. Remember, book one tells you how and why I adopted this practice from Dr. Lorraine Day.

My food intake is a rigid plan of action. Three full meals are required for optimum weight and nutrient achievements. My time for eating could vastly improve according to medical experts. Breakfast is usually eaten late morning, shifting the remaining two meals into late afternoon and night.

Usually, I don't encounter digestive or other difficulties. It is fear of knowing that medical recommendations say this is not good practice. The practice of eating as late as I do, particularly my last meal of the day, is not good. When I don't work a full day or on days off, my timing for eating is okay. You would think this might be the other way around, considering working requires eating. An unusual and opposite effect has always been a part of my eating patterns even when I worked for corporate America. This effect focuses on what you are doing at the time, then eat. Eating appears to be so enjoyable that way, work and get your special project out of the way. It is the sensation of saying to yourself, now food and me.

My position is that you must have aggressive plans, mentally physically, and spiritually. These plans help you launch and maintain a healthy lifestyle and fitness program for yourself.

Mental plans means conditioning your mind to accept the fact that you must perform the task that you set for yourself to do within a consistent cycle. That cycle can be daily, every other day or a standard variation built between expert recommendations and yourself. Dr. Cooper invoked another mind searching thought when he used the term "mind wellness." He stated that this term meant "keep your mind active, think positive thoughts and minimize the stress in your life."

Minimum, three times per week is the accepted norm by the health and fitness training gurus for exercise. These standards have been accepted by me since inception. An exercise attitude for me says exercise is a requirement, not an option. The goals established are reasonable and realistic. Further these goals are not too rigorous. Missing a planned day of exercise for me is the same as missing a planned doctor appointment. This required exercise mentality is a way of life for me. Exercise is not the sort of thing I dread doing each day of my established training cycle. It is something that I look forward to and enjoy the benefits exercise affords me mentally and physically. Further, the exercise sustains me until the next planned visit unless I deviate from the training cycle.

For me, it is a variety pack each daily cycle. That doesn't mean I don't perform the same tasks daily. My tasks vary widely but consistency keeps it place. Daily I walk and maintain a dance step routine on plastic steps achieving the goal to get exercise, air and sunshine on many days. Biking is every other day. Weight resistant training is every other day. Now that takes care of physical plans for me.

My spiritual cycle is maintained daily with devotional reading and prayer. The term "spirit wellness" was introduced to me by Dr. Cooper in this same UMM breakfast setting. This "spirit wellness" is the equivalent of spiritual lifestyle. The spirit must be constantly and consistently fed to attain optimum performance, he implied.

Launching a healthy lifestyle would not be complete without maintaining aggressive sleep and rest habits. These areas are mandated by a well maintained health and fitness program. Relaxation is a bonus piece added to my rest habits to achieve good results.

Easily I could get stuck in a rut and settle for just being able to work at peak levels and walk better. After all, this position I am in now is amiable compared to five and one half years ago. My passion for life and zeal to exceed what has already been accomplished doesn't let me stop and stay put. It is so gratifying to realize daily that God's favor accomplished this modern miracle for me. This daily attitude of gratitude is what keeps me pumping and reaching to get even better.

Daily, I keep trying to improve my walking ability and relieving myself of my left leg limp. You see multiple sclerosis' (m.s.) most notable outward sign to onlookers when I was first stricken was my left leg limp. There are days the limp is not as noticeable as others. That is the nature of m.s. You never know whether you are going to run at optimum level or below minimum from day to day. Many questions come from gym associates. It is a weekly toss up as to whether I get more questions from the gym or street people who see me frequently on my not so optimum days. These comments signal me about my progress to get better.

When my limp gives me a setback from time to time, I don't let disappointment stay with me long. Readily, I pick up the pieces and retool myself and efforts to get back on my journey to stay fit and healthy. Immense past efforts have brought comfort and peace knowing there is no pain associated with this limp. There was once a tingling sensation in my lower legs. This tingling felt like unwanted and undesirable spring sensations in my legs. This tingling feeling scared me as much as any other bad symptom of multiple sclerosis I experienced.

My Immune System and M.S. Five Years Later

It was the fear of not knowing where this tingling was leading my walking conditions and ability. As time progressed, my attitude to stick with plans to continue with an all natural approach to get better overall continued. Overall meant every inch of my body. Determination would not let me leave any part of my affected or unaffected body areas unprotected. That is, research through my own means continued along with medical visits with no known cure or relief from m.s. symptoms. During this research and trial period experienced by me, the suggested medical profession appeared to be single minded. The main methodology for m.s. symptom relief appeared to be the long term use of steroids with bad side effects.

A solution to the tingling came my way with the continued use of a particular gym machine. No matter where I went to use a gym, my legs and mental attitude led me to a leg press. Repeated use of this machine in my weekly gym cycles on an every visit basis created long lasting relief. Even traveling, I found this piece of gym equipment and its comforting effects.

This same determination never allowed me to give in to medications such as long term use of steroids to alleviate m.s. problems. Aside from the tingling in the lower leg areas, balance problems gets my vote for the second most fearful m.s. symptom I faced in my battle years with m.s. These balance problems kept me in a denial state for a lengthy time period. As people saw me stumbling or staggering, I used every excuse imaginable to get them off the subject as to why they saw me make that sort of move. My normal excuse was I stumbled over something in my way. Needless to say, there was usually little in my way. Most of the times it was a neatly unbuckled rug or the ground with no pebbles in the route.

My trainer/ friend gave me the gift of balance and coordination problem relief. He introduced and had special handmade steps for me to use during my workouts. After my ending term with him, I sought similar type of steps I could use on my own. The answer came when I discovered plastic tubular steps used by celebrities and fitness /dance experts on television. Quickly I was able to land a good set of plastic steps. These steps came with the tubular rings that I could build to my desired height. This proved to be the ultimate answer.

Use of these steps continue to negate my stumbling and staggering. Further techniques from gym dance experts continue to show me more improvement can be made through more consistent and additional aerobic exercises. When I experience the slightest off balance move, this is my trigger to let me know work is needed. This signal finds me racing to use the step routine on a two to three day cycle. In my early battle years with m.s., using the steps was a required daily function. Boredom and personal resistance set in. Therefore, I deviated from the daily to an as needed mostly basis. Sometimes, I find the energy and mindset to do this as part of my regular weekly workout .

Achieving walking longer distances without the left or right legs giving in to fatigue or discomfort reigns supreme. This solution has been achieved from constant use of gym weight resistant equipment targeting the leg muscles. Walking daily now is made possible and signals me when more gym exercise fuel is needed. The stationary bike adds range of motion to my legs and gives me a big boost to walk.

Realizing the achievements of a natural program to get better over time has firmly cemented my attitude. This attitude remains more improvement is ahead. Working with professionals and in this manner over time has shown me there is no quick fix to my left leg problem. My efforts and zeal to improve my leg through natural physical treatment and conditioning are intensified by past rewards. Courage and my never say die attitude has brought me 360 degrees from where I started. The joy brought daily from this attitude is knowing that my past attempts were not in vain. That gives me a burning desire to keep pushing harder and try new things that come with the wisdom of trials and research.

Self pity is down the corner from failure and quit. There is a huge cement block wall built some time ago that buffers me from that corner. That block wall took the same portions of attitude and faith Nehemiah embraced in rebuilding the walls around Jerusalem. Rev. Osteen said "years of faithful massive root system develops attitude undergrowth."

That undergrowth Rev. Osteen spoke about was woven into me through my grandfather's teachings (Papa Charlie, Dave). Those teachings instilled in me the will to complete all assignments the very best I can. That means giving all I have in achieving the desired results. You go beyond the call of duty to do what is expected. This attitude of gratitude is conveyed in every assignment approach and finalization.

Completing all assignments (business or personal) the very best that I can gives me a great sense of accomplishment. Each task or project as I call it gives me a chance to break it down and enjoy a mini success as I tread though stages of the assignment. Some might say that my stages are too slow or procrastination tactics. The benefits usually attained from acting in this manner outweigh the rush and get through approach.

An old job WCC acquaintance was hired in as a field auditor in my corporate America years. This acquaintance was a former junior college basketball coach and even had a decent game. Mike always made comments around me about "cream always rise to the top." One day I confronted him and asked him what did he mean by that old southern basketball coaching phrase. Mike couldn't stop laughing as he began to explain. He said "I always volunteer to be on your side for every project assigned in the office. The reason is that everyone in the office feels your job team and help are always going to outdo everybody else on assignments."

"You not only expect the best from everyone else but you show them how to do by example. You even wind up doing most of the work assigned yourself in cases. If anyone breaks down, you pick up the load or if anyone is ill or absent you are there in their place. Further, he said, have you ever seen cream in coffee or anything you put it in? It always rises to the top slowly but surely. Do you need more explanation was his final comment?"

Mike's comments can be better understood by WCC'S mentality. WCC (my former employer) always believed in competitive job performance incentive (rewards) programs. In order to accomplish goals it divided its office personnel into job teams with associated rewards programs attached. The entire company structure was similar including branch, region, and corporate levels.

It never occurred to look inside of myself until I was faced with Mike's explanation and analogy of me. After his assessment I did not know whether to feel good about me or just what. It sounded like I was perceived to be somewhat odd but a good odd.

Working in this manner as a self-employed person has proved to be extremely beneficial. People depend on you based on your work ethics and habits. These come natural and can't be taught quickly or easily.

Going that extra mile or beyond the call of duty (my grandfather's phrase) translates into an attitude of peace.

Tranquility and calmness engulf my thoughts and actions. Self confidence broadens with this attitude of peace. It recently occurred to me that Galatians 5: 22,23 had already captured the correct wording for this sort of self effort and character. "But the fruit of the Spirit is love, joy, peace, patience, kindness, goodness, faithfulness, gentleness and self- control."

Recently I was reminded by a living gentle giant to always leave time to reach out to someone else. In this lecture setting the giant said to the group "if you don't have one hour of time to spare away from your work to reach out to someone, then you are in the wrong job." The giant was signaling to the group to reach out to young people, our future, he reiterated. This living gentle giant capped his lecture by saying "the most important things in your life should be health, young people and family."

That is taken a step further by me daily in reaching out utmost to the young. Young people always inspire me to find ways to extend them a helping hand. There is another side of reaching out. That reaching out includes all the others. These others include someone who just needs a helping hand with a chore or car problem or financial assistance according to my own means. Sometimes along the way, I run across a person who just needs to sit down and talk.

Oftentimes, I am reminded that I can talk in big buckets and with substance. Other times, the person just needs someone to listen to their story or side. Oh, yes I can become the listener as well. That is one of the secrets of my professions, knowing when to talk and when to listen, both in big buckets. This attitude to help never leaves me without. Friendship and gratitude means the world to me

In my quest for optimum physical and mental performance I seek the full meaning and purpose of life. This meaning and purpose allows me to enjoy the privilege or reward given me to walk, talk and think. Gratefully, I seek to enjoy the privileges such as the beauty of nature. At the annual break of my profession's season, I take a getaway break to a completely nature oriented hideaway.

This hideaway has mountains, streams, lakes, golf courses, biking trails, tennis, basketball, beach and camping facilities. Supreme is the peace and tranquility. The community offers just about anything you could choose for fun and relaxation. Needless to say, I look forward to this break annually. At times I get urges from a friend, family member or my mate to sneak this visit in more than once per year. The community now has some nearby homes for sale. Their amenities are ideal for vacationing or planned retirement. That slip up was not supposed to get in this writing. Oh well, my well kept secret for years has already been uncovered by others.

Traveling has always been an artful past time for me. This reward was extended to me in my long-term corporate America endeavors. Daily travel was par for the course. It was not only a job requirement but a rich experience that took me far and near. This exposure allowed me to broaden my ideas and horizon. Many present day ideas have root connections to those travel experiences. Guess I'll have to resort to more travel in the near future to locate a new private spot.

CHAPTER 6

YOU COULD AND NEVER SHOULD TAKE THIS JOURNEY ALONE

Friends, associates and people whom I have met for the first time read my book one on multiple sclerosis and the immune system. Repeatedly, they have asked me what persuaded me to do all the research and many things I did. My answer was consistent. After listening to leading medical and nutritional experts on television and radio, I was convinced there was hope to get better using a total and committed natural approach. Their beliefs and methods were faith based.

This natural approach consisted of proper nutrition, exercise, sleep, rest, managing stress, and maintaining the right attitude. In the background of all the tools for success, faith in God persisted. Faith in God is the centerpiece for my every move to maintain my daily health, fitness, nutritional and spiritual lifestyles.

Spiritual lifestyle is a reward. It is a reward that you reap as you set out on the journey of life. This reward has been handed down from generation to generation. Rev. Joel Osteen describes it best as "being the beneficiary of deposits stored up by previous family members."

Rev. Osteen encourages us to make our own "deposits" for future generations to come with daily prayer and commitment to Christ. These deposits are created and made by your own daily actions. That is where these spiritual rewards come in handy. We can relate to helping others with difficult situations while trying to maintain our own situations.

Daily spiritual lifestyle's reward must be used daily. Like the adage goes, "if you don't use it, you'll lose it." You must exercise daily faith in your journey to get well and remain disease free. This exercise of faith goes beyond prayer and reading scriptures. You must act and trust in God with all your heart and mind. Good and rational decisions come from this trust.

Acting for me consists of never wavering with my daily exercise and nutritional habits. Sleep, rest and stress management are challenged daily. The key is how I pick up the pieces daily. When I stray off the course with sleep or rest, the remainder of my health and fitness management program is challenged. Centering my thoughts and feelings in Christ I become re-connected with my daily mission. Inner peace and serenity often result and affect my actions positively.

Stress management has been a consistent practice builder for me. Rarely, do I let a person or project detour me from daily personal or business goals and targets. When a rare uncontrollable detour is required I usually don't worry or fret fainthearted. Breaking things down into manageable parts has become a mainstay for me. Maintaining the right attitude is critical to all endeavors. Alternative implementation has become a way of life in my personal and business dealings.

My quest to maintain myself never goes without looking out for my fellow man. Always seizing the opportunity to help someone daily gives me a great deal of personal satisfaction. This help could be giving an encouraging word, allowing someone disabled to enter a door before me or assist them to cross the street, give a listening ear to someone who just wants you to listen to their personal or medical problems.

This journey of life was never designed to travel alone. Even when we attempt through trial and error to do everything on our own, we learn from our experiences life is not meant to do everything on our own. You should never take efforts with your own hands, mind and body to try and get well and maintain yourself. Daily prayer and devotion to God is required, not an option. God is my power source (fuel).

Each morning is begun by reading scripture. Each morning's words from such notable commentaries as Daily Bread, Daily Word or Upper Room encourage me to get up and get on with my walk, exercise program and work. Some days I pick up the bible and go back through the scriptures to get myself focused or revisit some important points a spiritual leader has made.

It is no magic that I walk without stumbling while taking a peaceful three fourth to one mile walk daily. Optimism and enthusiasm fill my body, mind and tank as I get on with the tasks, not work or chores to me. Three to four days per week my power source leads me to do more than walk. Biking, weight resistance training and aerobic conditioning come from this source.

My power source lights up my walk daily. Choosing the right exercise or the right combination of food daily becomes confusing at times. A mild setback or throwback of the past is usually the reason for this confusion. This setback or throwback can be in the form of an exercise challenge. It could be a challenge to lift a lower than normal amount of leg weights that normally sustain my daily conditioning. The setback or throwback could be nutritional. A particular food or drink could appear to take a mild condition in the opposite direction than what medical experts said that it would go. Sometimes fear, doubt, or drifting begins to set in my thoughts about mental or physical conditioning. Immediately, I race to my power source for answers through his holy word.

It has been times that I saw a person walking and I could not match that person's steps. Other times have allowed me to see a person walk a golf hole with such ease that I wondered why I could not do that with the same amount of effort and ease. That is where my power source quickly tunes me into how much faster I can walk or handle a chore than many other people. This sometimes comes in the form of assisting someone with a task or walking to pick up a playing partner's golf club.

Quickly, I am reminded that at one time the idea of walking a golf hole was no longer possible in my life. In fact, I had given up on the idea, of playing golf and even considered riding a scooter for the rest of my life off the golf course. Don't get me wrong, the scooter idea sounded like a good tradeoff. Envy sets in when I visit the local grocery store and see ladies and men wheel around with ease and joy in their mobile scooter counterparts. These people appear so peaceful, joyful and playful at times doing this.

Remindful, I sometimes engage in the thought that I was at one stage of this journey of life a robust and energetic specimen of a human being. Fear of a degenerative or any kind of major disease such as m.s. never entered my mind. This journey of life teaches and reaches. It reaches far beyond your own situation. During this journey I have met many with the same or similar degenerative illness I faced. Many had lost hope when I first saw them. There were others who shared my feelings and faith. This journey of life has allowed me to go full circle to return to a robust and energetic state daily. Some say "miracle cure" but I say daily walk with my power source.

Sad or negative thoughts come my way just as all human beings. These feelings are natural and one must acknowledge them as such. Critically important to me is that one must not allow these sad or negative moments to linger or consume them. For me, my thought process continues to move me higher and allows me to keep on pushing. My power source lets me know he is within me. Knowing this I keep myself calm, together and poised. It is with prayer that I acknowledge God's presence. Prayer sustains my every motive and move. Prayer puts me on the right side of the track allowing me to surge forward. As a result sad, negative and hurtful thoughts seem to disappear in mid air.

These tracks of life let me know that I have been equipped with all of the right tools to stay fit and healthy physically and spiritually. There is no reason for doubt when you reach this pinnacle in your walk with Christ. Trials and tribulations are great teachers for me. Daily living experiences challenge me but point me to the next course of action. Overcoming challenges is par for the course.

God's favor is a gigantic spiritual reward. This favor is God's way of showing you he has control of your life, health and plans for you to follow him. The key is for you to accept this favor by expressing your belief. If your challenge is physical illness, this belief is that you can get well by following God's plan for your life daily. The key is daily and not random or when you want to do it. This is the same with exercise, nutritional and sleep habits, attitude and managing daily stress.

Understanding the importance of my faith keeps me focused and my thoughts flowing in the right direction. Rev. Osteen called this faith in God "quiet confidence." Many times in this journey of life circumstances have caused me to reconsider whether or not I was on the right road. Business deals have soured at times when funds seemed their lowest. This "quiet confidence" allowed me to rise above circumstances and further showed me I was already loaded with the artillery I needed to accomplish my goals. There was no reason to sit there stuck in the mud and cry out, why me? Instead, each time I was able to realize the situations put me in better position by showing me to swim harder and faster.

It is faith that guides my actions, moves and steps in my business dealings. Faith shows me when the road is clear for me to make a decision and take a detour off the normal route. In other words, many times in business or personally, I must take a riskier course than normal.

Faith has been monumental in all my decisions regarding dealing with m.s. In my early decisions regarding therapy, faith led me to good physician treatment. Along the way, faith showed me that eventually the medical drug treatment initially prescribed and used for at least three years would wear out my liver. This meant an early or premature fatality for me. This same faith led me to do over eighteen months of research. Faith proved to be the eventual right answer enabling me to get off the prescribed medication. It allowed me to use a natural approach to get better and remain healthy.

This natural approach remains in use today. Only a spiritual reward through God's favor could have led me to do the research and choose the correct material without any medical background. Further God's favor shows me daily to continue with the same daily tools I began with five years ago. These tools are enhanced with time and change to God given (favor) to other men and women. This change could be in the use of gym equipment, nutritional habit suggestions or physician recommendations.

My faith walk with Christ many times allow me to mentally reflect. Reflections go back to some of the gentle giants in memory I saw handle their spiritual rewards. These reflections give me reassurance and allows me to use them as my own steppingstones. One would readily think I am referring to family members only. This is not the case in my life. True, family members have been extremely crucial steppingstones for me. These family members cemented my foundation and plotted my life course. However, the many lessons learned and wisdom gained have come from the many events in my life. Each gentle giant in memory taught me something about life and myself.

After leaving home for collegiate life, I arrived in a large city in which I knew absolutely no one. There were no relatives nor friends to even set up a chat line with, just me. College life and that back home family member foundation took care of that. No one was ever a stranger. Three college professors took special interest in me and steered me to heights I could not envision alone. One such giant in memory was Vera Benton, a communications professor. Ms. Benton took me by the hand and placed me in classes she taught for two years (at least four semesters of successful work). To this day I am gratified of the efforts she put into me. Her efforts boosted me to reach levels and heights of achievement in the business world (corporate and private practice). These efforts are further exhibited in my achievement levels in professional examinations, public speaking and communicating with my fellow man.

Professor Willie Richardson was an Accounting professor and practicing CPA who spotted me in my freshman year and assisted me in choosing my college curriculum. Mr. Richardson introduced me to the college business department head, Mr. Oscar Burnett. Mr. Burnett told Mr. Richardson he was responsible for me. After hearing this, I grew apprehensive because I didn't understand that statement. Each semester I began to understand that statement Mr. Burnett had made. Mr. Richardson was tougher on me than many of my classmates. Having grown up in this manner under my grandparents I readily understood his approach.

In my junior year, Mr. Burnett and Mr. Richardson entered one other student and myself in a special IRS sponsored program. The program involved one-half semester classroom participation with the IRS and one half work with neighborhood work centers preparing individual taxes. How little did we know that this program would later become known nationally as the IRS' VITA program. That program has been expanded nationally and is alive today.

Recently, I read an article on an Atlanta legend who entered my life in the late 1990's as a gentle giant. This gentle giant now in memory was Mr. James Paschal. After conversing with Mr. James for about the third time I was always curious as to why he often sought to converse with me on business matters. Also, I was equally curious as to why he was always so complimentary of me and my work habits. He even compared me to he and his brother's work habits and ethics.

Later, I found through a local banker that my previous college instructor, CPA Willie Richardson, was this giant's business Accountant prior to moving out of the city.

Needless to say, this giant's comments are engraved on my chest. The span I knew the giant was short compared to many who had been around this giant and his brother during their original business venture days. However, I have some un regrettable and unforgettable soul filled memories of my short time with him. Also, I have collector items such as signed Christmas cards, thank you notes and at least one special invitation to an event honoring him and his brother he personally delivered to me. These were either given directly to me by him personally or directed through his personal assistant to get them to me annually. Even when I moved away from the initial office building where he met me, he told his assistant to keep up with me.

After undergraduate work I was fortunate to join the ranks of fortune 100 Westinghouse Credit Corporation (WCC). This part of my journey was made possible by the vote of Vice- President Ben Russell, who transferred to Pittsburgh as Vice –President of WCC simultaneous with my hiring at the local Atlanta branch level. On his precious few visits back to Georgia he often sought to find me and speak to me one on one. Mr. Russell even came back to give me my first major company award during my first year of WCC service. He often would say to me during his visits "one day, Joe, you are coming to Pittsburgh with me to see the Falcons and Steelers" Mr. Russell knew I had become fond of football while in college and even went to college with a standout Falcon.

Mr. Russell didn't let me down. During the infamous Steel curtain dynasty, Mr. Russell arranged for me to come to Pittsburgh on company business. He gave me four Steelers football tickets. This same team won that year's Super Bowl and the next year also. The tickets were great, forty yard line in the old Three Rivers Stadium.

It was so gratifying to receive the tickets for an October game. Weather checks and all other preplanning things were done to make this a successful week long joint game-business trip. I even packed the heaviest winter coat I owned, a Columbo style trench coat that was pretty classy with a heavy lining for Atlanta winters. Half time of that football game, my guests (all WCC southern statesman) and I left as it was too cold for us to handle the weather. The Pittsburgh fans laughed at us as we left. These fans were bear chest and appreciative of Pittsburgh winters. This was real football weather to them but it wasn't even funny to us. The score nor great players of that day meant very little to us as we left.

As I continued my journey with WCC, I entered into managerial ranks. During this period I teamed up with three great individuals who became my daily friends. Friends in the business world usually means regular lunch pals or occasional night out with family. These three individuals created lifelong friendships with me. True it all started in the office working side by side in one of these individual's case. This individual, Sam Bryant, was just like many of the other gentle giants that entered my life in Atlanta. Sam was determined to keep our friendship growing.

After introducing me to his wife and daughters, he put his best friend, Chuck Grad who lived in a neighboring state, together with me. Chuck, Sam and I began expanding our relationship with regular visits to each person's residential city. Sam was a University of Alabama alumni and Chuck was a Pennsylvania product. Sam saw me on more than one occasion reading about the legacy of Bear Bryant from Alabama. Sam made it possible for the three of us to go to a University of Alabama game while Coach Bryant was still coaching. Yes, I got a chance to see the famous Bear Bryant's lean on the goal post while the players went through pre game routines.

During our many visitations to sporting events and entertainment sites, Chuck and Sam even went to one of my small school's (MBC) basketball games. Our friendship didn't just stop at attending sporting events. Sam and Chuck were good friends and frequent golf partners with our Regional Operations manager, Hoover Keith. Hoover had asked for my services in his department on more than one occasion but I never left the District level to the Regional office. Since Atlanta housed a Regional office it gave me opportunities to visit and have lunch on a frequent basis with Mr. Keith. This group of three plus me formed a regular foursome golf partnership that expanded for years to come.

These three gentle giants not only taught me the game of golf from scratch but gave me my first set of golf clubs. After giving me the clubs, they told me that when I got good enough I would buy my own. Boy, did I laugh inside. There was no excuse to keep me off any course. We played the likes of Mystery Valley, Sugar Creek, Pine Isle, Callaway Gardens, San Destin and many more in four states. Golf grew from frustration to a weekly fun filled event for me.

These three giants somehow knew my competitive nature would escalate me to learn and enjoy the game on a higher level one day. They were right. Golf became a craze of mine right away. Eventually I took a job on the road with WCC. This allowed me to play golf frequently with business clients and practice, practice, practice. Reading golf magazines for tips and practicing at driving ranges on the road sent my game to favorable competitive levels. Sam, Chuck and Hoover began pairing me with other golf associates with good competitive games.

WCC clients noticed my improvement and began inviting me to golf tournaments. This led to big events with professional sponsors such as Sony and Amana. In addition I was able to go to leading pro tournaments and see players on the PGA tour play. All of this propelled my journey of life and filled me with life long memories. Oh, I bought that set of golf clubs tailored and specially fitted for me. These were designed and crafted by a previous out of town tour player. The irons are ping style and still in use today.

Aside from golf I maintained my personal life with friends and family. One gentle giant now in memory that stood out in my personal journey was a friend, Herman Lewis (Bo). Bo was older than me but kept his eyes on me. Bo was a local plumber who was good. He was so good in his profession that leading companies would always call him in for major problems. Bo was cited by a leading businessman as the "Joe Lewis of his profession." Echoing that caption, I even recall a major water main break on the north side of Atlanta, over thirty miles from where Bo worked and resided. Bo was called in on that major city and county problem. Bo even was listed as the lead on the Jackson prison installation, Jackson, Georgia. Great work ethics and family were his drivers.

When I had a special plumbing line problem that had lasted for years, it was Bo that told me when it was time to replace the entire line. He even mapped out his strategic plan and had me do the preparatory work such as calling the gas company to mark the line. To this day I remember the fright in my heart and mind wondering how I was going to raise the money to pay for such a big project as replacing an entire sewer pipe line. Bo did it for one third of the cost of two major companies that I had come out and it worked as he designed. Bo didn't cut any corners. He strategized like all giants, Joe Lewis, Michael Jordan, and Bill Gates. He knew exactly how he was going to do it but his approach emulated those other giants. He brought in huge equipment that roared and rumbled through the entire neighborhood street. Neighbors came out of their homes on a late Saturday evening to see what earthquake was going through their yards. You don't leave a giant like that off your team.

You could never recapture the gentle spirit of my grandfather, Dave (Papa Charlie), now a gentle giant in memory. This man instilled in me many manly characteristics with his kind and gentle mannerism on a daily basis. His many wisdom filled chats helped build my vocabulary. Papa Charlie's gift of numbers from his profession as an Artisan well builder spilled over into me. That was no accident. His determination to give me his gift made that possible.

Papa Charlie regularly took me shopping one on one for clothing and shoes. He had some mean threads himself. When I left for college I took some of his double breasted sports jackets that had come back in style. Coordinating them with new slacks caused some of my college classmates to tell me they were sharp and even asked where did I buy them. Patience and determination were two of his undeniable traits. These quickly became traits I marveled and sought after.

A gentle giant in memory who not only steered me in the right direction in my early years of life was my Godmother, Susie Moore "Mama Sue." Mama Sue was a well educated guidance director in the local school system in the State of Georgia. Mama Sue entered my life through Mama in the AME church. She carried me on many of her routes in the county neighborhood for me to witness her in action. Normally, I did not enter the houses on the visits with her but it was so eye opening to see the kinds of conditions she drove up to. Her specialty was youth school compliance and enforcement. Quickly I gained knowledge of her skills as she embraced me to pump wisdom into my head.

Financially, she gave me work assignments around her residence she knew I could handle to earn any dollars. No money was given to me unless I earned it first was an unwritten rule between us. This produced strong work ethics and behavior in me. Never did I shortcut any work assigned. Every effort was given on anything she gave me to do. My best foot was always put forward.

Mama's Sue house needed painting badly, inside and outside. A couple of local painters had invested a two year period of time teaching me their trades. This included outside and inside painting techniques. Their work took me all over my small hometown in various neighborhoods. These painters, Louie Brown and Homer Burch were well known to the community and produced very good work results in neighboring towns. Mama Sue was inspired by the work I had done at two nearby homes for one of these painters. As a result she allowed me to paint her home, as in main residence. Trust me I didn't let her down and even contracted one of these painter/teachers to round out my loose ends.

Even after high school, Mama Sue followed me to college and visited me regularly at a familiar site near campus, Paschal's Restaurant. You know I never remember being late for any of her 200 mile plus visits. Many of the visits were coordinated with state business and yet others were to see her "God son" one on one. Her wisdom and ethics carry on in my life today.

Oftentimes, I am reminded of two gentle spiritual, wisdom filled giants in memory that appeared early in my life. These were my Grandmother, "Mama" Essie Mae and her sister, Mary. Both giants resembled each other in appearance, spirit and mannerism. The main difference was age. Aunt Mary was younger and was always eager to take me by the hand and show me the ropes. Aunt Mary instilled in me entrepreneurial spirit and burning desire to succeed daily. No matter what trial or tribulation came my way Aunt Mary gave me the blue print to tackle it with her wisdom.

Her calm approach to handling any obstacle, challenge or chore fit Mama's profile like a twin sister. Therefore, I enjoyed the many days spent with Aunt Mary when she sent for me. Quietly and patiently, these sisters developed determination in me to emulate themselves. Aunt Mary always gave me small carpentry and other sundry jobs in and outside her home. These included floor joists and wall panels, gathering eggs from chickens, and sowing seeds in vegetable and fruit gardens. You can imagine the chore tasks didn't keep me eager to come by Aunt Mary's.

You see Aunt Mary had highly fashionable clothing tastes. These tastes were detected by several young members of the family. However, I worked my way into Aunt Mary's heart. She physically showed me how to shop for clothes after finishing my chores on a regular basis. Weekly shopping for ties, tie pins, matching and well coordinated ascots, cuff links, shirts, pants and sports coats started with Aunt Mary. These sisters never expressed jealousy, just respect and love for each other and their families.

Mama often echoed Aunt Mary's wisdom advice on a daily basis. This let me know who was the elder and how it all started. Mama usually taught by example. One of her examples that has always remained in front of my life was the story of Joseph.

This story is captured in Genesis, Chapters 37 through 50. Mama constantly reminded me to read the story of Joseph in Genesis. Later I began to catch on to Mama's motive for the reminders. These reminders appeared whenever I came to her with feelings of being done wrong or felt sorry for myself. Also, if I felt overwhelmed by thinking I had done too much in "God's eyes," this reminder came up. This "victim of circumstance" mentality quickly eroded with prayer and meditation. Trust me, it still works today.

As I grew from childhood to man hood, the story of Joseph stayed with me. Comfort and calm stems from this story, and it is equally rewarding to hear ministers deliver sermons from these scriptures. Rev. Charles Stanley captured the entire story of Joseph in one of his 2008 telecasts.

Some living gentle giants enter and remain in my life today. Critical to my success is to listen to and observe their actions. It is with understanding that I accept these giants as spiritual rewards from God. God's favor many times is clearly demonstrated through their words of wisdom or actions. The ability to discern comes from reading God's word and listening to his messengers. King Solomon's Proverbs are powerful rewards that define the ability to discern.

Also critical in my spiritual lifestyle is consistency in every phase of my plan to maintain good health. Daily, I am urged to read and search God's word. This reading illuminates my daily path personally and business wise. Reading many times shows me how other "soldiers" I admire take their faith walk. In 2008, I picked up one of my daily commentaries and found an article on Robin Robins, a nationally television personality. Robin had written a book about her life and battle with a degenerative disease.

What was more interesting to me was channeling my energy to mentally review Robin's early entry into my life. Robin was a local Atlanta sports show personality prior to going nationally. She also had been a very good athlete. Immediately, her story was of interest for me to read.

My spiritual lifestyle is enhanced by my ability to share my medical successes with others verbally when I feel the need arises. Selectively, I handle opportunities to share this sort of information. Usually, the opportunity arises from talking to an acquaintance in the gym, grocery store, occasional visit to retail outlets, business meeting or travel. Engaging in friendly conversations about mutual lifestyles, you find yourself sharing knowledge about what you do to maintain yourself. Most times this becomes a rewarding experience.

Through all of my past physical challenges, I have attained wisdom and guidance from my power source. This wisdom has sparked remarkable recovery from a disease that threatened to take me out of the work force and walking. Mentally, this disease would have subdued my thoughts and plans for every aspect of my life.

The words of Andre Crouch say it best "To God Be The Glory For The Things He Has Done. With His Blood He Has Saved Me. With His Power He Has Raised Me. To God Be The Glory."

CHAPTER 7
TEN YEARS LATER WITH MY LIMP

Mentally and physically now, I am learning to change and adapt to the seasons of business (work) and the seasons of the year (nature). During the first four months of the year I realize that it is an abnormally busy work season for me. An early morning start is required to do everything for each day of this season. This avoids panicky and rushing situations throughout the day. The mindset is smoother and most of the day I find myself cruising through the day. Work projects appear easier and less demanding to get done. Solutions appear that may have hid themselves in prior attempts to resolve.

During the first four months, my exercise routines must not stop. The same vigor applies during this period as in the rest of the year. Adapting and changing I have learned to take advantage of the early morning get up time. Walking is usually everyday. For the past two years I have missed less than twenty days per year walking. This walk fits better in the early morning before I get into my exercise routine or get started with business (work). The walk most days occurs near home. While traveling out of town on business or pleasure, the walk is not neglected. A suitable walking site is usually located during a pre screen ride while entering a new locale.

An outdoor site is usually my goal. This gives me a three in one advantage doctors frequently talk about, **air, exercise and sunshine**. The natural **air** surrounds me without doing a thing but walking. Natural air gets the lungs and bronchial systems pumping.

Exercise is obtained as part of the natural process of walking. Even though I feel the refreshment and energy given to me from walking, I don't put exercise to the forefront as the reason I walk. By that I mean I don't use exercise for walking as a replacement for my required gym activities.

On many days I am able to meet the **sunshine**. Sunshine in Atlanta is not a rarity. This sunshine stated in more than one medical publication "triggers our bodies to make vitamin D."

Recent research is on going on the significance and role of vitamin D and multiple sclerosis. One study reported from the Harvard School of Public Health suggested "that higher levels of vitamin D found in participants' bodies decreased the risk for developing multiple sclerosis later in life." The same study authors were "careful to point out that the study does not prove that increasing vitamin D levels will decrease your risk for developing multiple sclerosis."

Even though there is no certainty of vitamin D's role with m.s there is more surety of its roles with bones. Vitamin D is known as a strong bone builder. Strong bones are needed for every physical thing I do. M.S. patients are known as frequent fallers. This was truly the case for me in my early battle years with m.s. No bone break was experienced by me with my many falls in previous years. Discussions often come up on why I didn't encounter bone problems. Quick to point out, frequent walking and my food choices had to be the core reasons that supported me.

EverydayHealth.com continues to post some interesting multiple sclerosis subjects. A latter 2009 internet posting read "According to the Partners' Multiple Sclerosis Center, multiple sclerosis has a higher incidence in North America, southern parts of Australia, and northern Europe, suggesting that the farther you live from the equator, the greater your risk for developing multiple sclerosis."

"Does this mean you should pack up and move to a warmer climate? Not necessarily. The link between vitamin D, known as the sunshine vitamin, and m.s. could explain why areas closest to the equator typically have the lowest rate of multiple sclerosis. Research indicates that vitamin D, which the human body generates in response to sunlight, may play some role in protecting against m.s. It has yet to be determined whether taking vitamin D supplements might carry the same benefit as exposure to sunlight appears to do. If you already take vitamin D supplements, you can be confident in the benefits that experts do know about, Vitamin D helps boost the immune system function and may aide the body in absorbing calcium."

A huge lift is present when I am able to get this three in one from walking outside (air, exercise and sunshine). Weather conditions sometimes play havoc on my morning walk outside. Pre – planning comes into place to either try a pm walk or seek an inside walking spot. While in town, I have a gym spot with an inside track. Out of town efforts are go with the flow.

After the initial four months of the year, my challenge to walk daily is not as a big of a struggle the remainder of the year. It isn't even a secondary thought to miss a day of walking during the May through December months. Even seasonal changes don't limit my walking time and distance. It pays big dividends that Georgia usually has mild winter conditions.

Throughout the entire twelve months I feel and see a huge difference now in my ability to walk more comfortably daily. Falls and stumbling have stopped completely. Balance is the single most improved symptom I notice myself without friends, co-workers or clients who notice me bring to light. My improved balance affects my walks positively and there is no more stop and catch myself from fear of a fall due to balance problems.

Carefulness is still a big part of my game plan. Going up and down stairs, I am not ashamed to hold on to rails and proceed gingerly in my walking pace. Sporting events seem to always be in venues with steps that challenge me mentally and physically. However, I haven't made a false move yet in this sort of atmosphere.

Stiff joints have stopped during fall and winter months. There are no colds nor sniffling during all four seasons. My fourth and fifth years of consistently staying with my ten step mostly natural plan revealed the changes in stumbling, falls and stiff joints. Previously lack of falls and no colds had told me I was on the right track to getting better.

Walking each a.m. for me is comfortable and not painful. You can't see yourself, your posture nor whether or not you appear in pain or uncomfortable to onlookers. Questions all the time from people let me know that my walk is not as fluid as it once was. I must appear in pain to some judging from the types of questions. Questions such as was I involved in a car accident, is it knee or hip problems? Apparently the m.s changes the appearance to onlookers of the problem.

One lady who regularly meets me in the a.m. walk route asked me in 2009 if I had considered herbal supplements. This walk with this lady began about three months prior to her comments. She even had the name and address from a GNC store she had visited. On and on she went to sell me on her idea about the supplements. After she finished I told her the limp was started with m.s. Also, I told her about my research and why I walk and workout. She was blown away when I let her employ a manual strength test I regular engage in with people. Thank goodness that ended the questionnaire periods from her and other nosy neighbors.

A big reason I venture out to walk early in the mornings is to walk alone. This gives me full enjoyment of the gift of walking that has been restored to me after a bout with m.s. Also, a big reason I enjoy early am workouts is to avoid a party and visitation appearance. This is similar to uninvited gym guests in between your sets of gym equipment use. It is so rewarding to do my daily workout and walk alone. There are times I am invited to workout with a friend, co – worker or mate. When this happens I readily accept the opportunity and my mindset is different. It becomes a fun experience participating and sharing with someone. The sharing is most gratifying.

Early morning walking daily and stationary biking are my core components for aerobic workout activity. Stationary biking alternates between a daily workout or bi-daily workout. This choice is aimed at preventing boredom. An occasional free style ride achieves the same purpose but adds a little more fun. The problem now is I have got to buy me a new bike. My old bike was given to a younger friend recently who had no bike but desired to stay fit.

Biking has been a part of my entire five and one half year plan. However, it wasn't until year five that I began to make a concentrated effort to do the bike daily similar to the walk. During the first four months of the year flexibility is key. Early morning is optimum time to do the biking. Sometimes during the first four months, that is not realistic. The bike ride usually doesn't occur until the after work evening hours.

Again, the mindset remains, get the biking in. Biking accomplishes two major things for me. It allows the legs to swing like a pendulum, free flowing movement. This movement gives me confidence that I have control over my ability to walk without stumbling. Thrusting forward I feel power in the movement of the legs. Momentum is gained with each step after a good ten minute plus bike ride. Secondly, the mental reward of knowing that I have done something to help my cardiovascular system. A prime advantage is targeting the heart rate tracked on my bike.

It is of great concern to me to watch the vital signs medical professionals check most. These include blood pressure and the target heart rate. Either of these signs not on point signal me to search for answers as to what is not happening or what am I doing wrong. The normal tendency is to check for lack of effort or am I doing enough time and distance. Biking gives me good anticipated vital sign numbers. This gives me confidence when I walk into my doctor's office for regular checkups. Most times I have not been disappointed during my five and one half year stretch. However, the disappointed visits get me searching and researching until the problem is fixed, better and stable numbers.

There was a period of about three weeks I experienced higher than normal pressure readings. The readings were discovered during a regular check up visit. The doctor's nurse nor I had no idea nor suspicion that my blood pressure readings had increased. She made the statement after the reading that the numbers were not seriously out of range. That just made me boil inside to myself at me, not her. Searching for answers from within and reading began to discover what I had done wrong in the short few weeks to cause my blood pressure reading to get in the red zone. The red zone for me is out of the healthy range for physician readings.

After about three days of self searching it occurred to me that exercise couldn't possibly be the culprit. Walking and gym activities had not slowed during this period. The frequency and pace had been on track during this period. Tracing my steps back to eating told me I had drifted away from the valuable omega three on a regular basis. Instead I had replaced it with a substitute favorite that was not omega three contents but a good food choice. Omega three and garlic are known in the medical community for their blood pressure reduction assistance. Sure enough just a few days change of diet prior to my next regularly planned check up reading gave me decreased readings. Most importantly was the mental anxiety relief.

Even though I survived that scare, another valuable lesson was learned. Daily I must get back on my good health goals and stick with them in order to remain intact.

Combination exercise routines are maintained at optimum levels to ensure quality health and desired good health numbers. Utmost to heart health maintenance is aerobic conditioning.

Joseph L. Wilson

REGULAR AEROBIC EXERCISES IN USE TODAY CONSISTS OF-

WALKING

STATIONARY BIKING

STEP EXERCISES

STRENGTH TRAINING EXERCISES IN REGULAR USE TODAY CONSISTS OF-

LEG PRESS MACHINES

LEG LIFTS

LEG CURLS

CALF RAISE MACHINES

ABDOMINAL MACHINES

SEATED DIP MACHINES

LATERAL ARM RAISE MACHINES

PECTOROID FLY MACHINES

ARM CURLS WITH FREE WEIGHTS

FLEXIBILITY EXERCISES IN REGULAR USE TO DAY CONSISTS OF-

FLOOR EXERCISES

SINGLE LEG RAISES

SIDE LEG RAISES

QUAD STRETCHES

STEP EXERCISES

Next order of business for my daily goals is maintenance of my **nutritional goals**. This whale of a goal is as big as exercise. That is, it requires a great deal of time and commitment each day to maintain. Achieving lesser than expected good vital numbers has shown me a correlation between diet and exercise. Most of the times my numbers were not on point during the five and one half year stretch, diet was the culprit. In order for readers to better understand me I should rephrase one of the above statements. My diet and me were the culprits, not diet alone.

Most times when I received a not so favorable vital sign report, I was able to trace the problem. It was not only what I ate but the regularity that I kept piling it on. Many times I refused to let a certain food choice get past me during a weekly cycle. It was not uncommon that I ate the lesser desired food choice two to three times per week. Even though this lesser desired food choice was a good food choice, the preparation was the problem, fried and too much sodium content.

It is not an easy nutritional lifestyle that I maintain. Good food and liquid choices are musts for me to remain healthy and disease free. Further it is so hard for me to maintain the required three good food choice full meals per day. My friends and family ridicule me more than anyone. Phrases such as "I won't eat that sort of food for breakfast to I can't eat that way" constantly ring in my head. My lunch size and food choice is the latest poster child picked on by this same group.

My daughter can't wait to tell people how and where I usually eat for lunch. Even though she has this run and tell that mentality about my food choices she regularly follows suit. She hasn't directly and openly admitted it to me but she eats that way most times now. Her realization of the good health benefits are reason enough. How do I know about her eating habits as of late ? Guess who pays for lunch most days?

Even more difficult for me are holiday lifestyle habits. Holiday lifestyle habits one, two and three (exercise, food water and juice) can't be left at home alone, You must pack them with you when traveling is the holiday choice. This four in one bunch is difficult at home daily but traveling adds challenge. Adding this challenge to my luggage requires much organization to get them in properly. You can't just squeeze in this much bulk and muscle. Carefully pre-planning my trip and route (s) I begin shopping and packing early. Last minute packing presents failure.

Having shopped and packed I usually feel energized enough to start my trip. Car travel is more suitable to my tasks ahead because of the flexibility afforded. Air or other means of travel means more planning techniques and exercising patience.

Home holiday choices pose bigger challenges sometimes than traveling away. You have visitors, friends and family with their special requests for food and drink that you must accommodate. This is not a compromise issue. You just simply can't expect anyone else to do what you do for your lifestyle habits.

There is the added chore of entertaining inquisitive friends and family member questions about your eating habits. It may be better to limit your answers to questions about your liquid intake (drinking) habits especially during holiday festivities. There is the age old question, "Why don't you eat or drink this with me just this one time?"

My **good food choices** are shown in the following charts that I have labeled as my favorite foods by meal type.

MY BREAKFAST MEAL CHOICE I EAT THE MOST PER DAY

LARGE BOWL OATMEAL WITH PARSLEY (honey or raisin or strawberries as toppings)

HONEY WHEAT BREAD BUNS (usually two bun sizes)

ONE BANANA

ONE RED APPLE

ONE LARGE CUP GRAPES

ONE BOWL STRAWBERRIES

MY LUNCH MEAL CHOICE I EAT THE MOST PER DAY

COLLARDS

CORN

SWEET POTATOES OR YAMS

GREEN BEANS OR LIMA BEANS

SLICED TOMATOES (about two slices per meal)

1 VEGGIE EGG ROLL

MY DINNER FOOD CHOICES
I EAT THE MOST

ORIENTAL STYLE ALMOND FRIED CHICKEN

BROWN RICE

STEAMED BROCCOLI IN OYSTER SAUCE

VEGGIE OR SPRING ROLL

OR

VEGETABLE GARDEN SALAD MEDLEY (consisting of spinach, lettuce, tomatoes, carrots, cucumbers, honey mustard dressing from good health provider)

CHIPS (good health provider) or baked potato

SUPPLEMENTS I USE THE MOST

PARSLEY

GARLIC

ROSEMARY

THYME

OLIVE OIL

HONEY

BARLEY

ALMONDS

SNACKS I EAT THE MOST DAILY

FRUIT SNACKS INCLUDE GRAPES, PLUMS, PEACHES, SLICED MELONS WHEN IN SEASON

NUTS SUCH AS PEANUTS, PECANS, ALMONDS, WALNUTS

POTATO CHIPS, POPCORN

WHEAT CRACKERS

CHART ON MY DAILY LIQUID INTAKE

WATER (early am usually before morning walk)

JUICE (early am before breakfast)

WATER (early pm before lunch)

WATER (later pm after lunch and before dinner)

JUICE (later pm before dinner)

You might note that my **liquid intake** has changed significantly since my inception to get well. Changes were made as I continued to progress better and better. Also, a series of bladder infections caused me to change my approach and liquid intake. Urologist help was sought in this process. This has not detracted from my efforts to stay disease free but my daily consistency is required..

It is worth noting that I bought me a juicer, top of the line in 2009. The purchase of the juicer altered my number of eight ounce glasses per day from three to maximum two. Most days I am able to maintain the standards of the above chart. The juicing is done 100% of the time from home. Juicing naturally this way comes with a big cleanup tag and preparation time.

The refreshing and energized feeling natural juicing gives me is worth the preparation and cleanup time. Juices bought from the store gave me a huge advantage for almost five years. No cleanup tag and the added advantage of the producers implementing the right proportions of natural ingredients. Added to that was the fact that these producers apparently had impeccable research team members on board. This could be gauged by the vitamin and other benefits advertised in their sales promotions and labels. Further research by me supported their positions.

Today juicing naturally creates more research on my part to gauge my vitamin and good nutrition intake. Surprisingly, this was not a big transition for me. It was fairly smooth in that the juices I use require many of my natural daily diet intake. The cost to me has not appeared to be an increase because of my liquid and food lifestyle. The store juices were quite costly. It appears to be an even trade or more cost effective way for me to buy my ingredients to do my own juicing.

On the other hand, my water intake has remained steady. Getting three eight ounce glasses per day in does not constitute a wrestling match. Rarely, do I exceed this self-established maximum because I feel full after topping out at three glasses of water per day. It agrees with my nutritional goals and bladder problems experienced in late 2008 and mid 2009. Good urology strategy helped significantly with this change in total liquid diet intake. It took a strong second opinion from a second urology group to get me back on track. More than a second opinion, the group changed the medical strategy. This sent me reeling for research on how to adapt the liquid intake to a sound level. The level meant no loss of nutritional intake from juicing and water.

The new strategy has worked for over six successive months. It gives me good nutrition which maintains sound energy levels. Most important to note is that no other medical flare up of any sort has occurred. It took the expertise of two different urologist teams and my internist to get me on track. This area is not being tossed aside. My team of medical providers have me on six month health watch.

Today my hours of work and sleep are changed from the original rehab period. Now my normal work hours begin after my workout and walk. Rarely is it necessary for me to use a super early hour start time to begin work projects. This start time was mandatory during my rehab years. Now I have options and I only use an earlier than the announced office hours when peak season or projects dictate.

Individual work stock pile signal me to make adjustments. This affects our business mostly during the tax season period. Occasional needs for some auxiliary services and post tax season services get top heavy at times. During other periods of the year, I am just as busy but the character of the work demand is different. Corporate work and case work require longer and sustained periods of work emphasis on each account. Consistency is the critical key to all of our work habits and projects.

A typical day for me is no where complete today without the unity of **sleep, rest and relaxation**. This ever present threesome round out my day. The day sometimes is a busier than normal work day or a day filled with big demands. Drive to get the work done to high quality levels puts me in position to look forward to joining the big three later.

My sleep, rest and relaxation lifestyle is an immense boost to my personal side. Further, increased energy and alertness open the door daily for increased work productivity. Planning and awareness of side issues receive better attention by me daily. The big three impacts that greatly.

Stressful events despise me as much as I despise them. Television watching is carefully scrutinized. Mostly comedy oriented and sporting events consume my television watching. Even the dance contests and programs are back on my agenda big time. The election of a new President has created interest in more news events. The stock channel, headline and CNN channels are back on my daily to do list. These areas are required for me to stay abreast of what I do for a daily living for clients and myself. Information seeking is my goal, not soaking in stressful events.

Choice and alternative planning are key ingredients for successfully managing stress for me. Choosing and deciding work great with communication. When I don't want to do something I usually communicate that to the asking party quickly to avoid ill feelings. More eventful activities are on my agenda. This includes sporting events, visiting friends, acquaintances, church activities, golf and volunteer work. Leisure and nature oriented activities occupy more of my time these days.

When the big three (sleep, rest and relaxation) are not around, I crave walking for pleasure in a nature environment. This can be alone or preferably with my mate to share the thoughts of the moments. My spirit is fed greatly with this nature environment and mentality. Mentally it is so refreshing and nourishing to share the simple things of life we take for granite. My faith is many times restored to witness nature's courses.

Speaking of faith, you may recall that torch of faith passed on from PAPA CHARLIE, my grandfather to MAMA, my grandmother to me in chapter six of book one. Well, it has appeared to me in my daily relationships, my youngest sibling is reaching for that torch from me. She is being assisted by a more than capable former state track champion, her partner and first cousin from childhood to adulthood. Together I don't think they'll miss it when I release.

RECOMMENDED READING LIST

Harvard Men's and Women's Health Watch, Harvard Medical School

Harvard Medical Special Health Report Series, Harvard Medical School

Men's Health Advisor, Cleveland Clinic

Mayo Clinic Health Letter, Mayo Clinic Health Solutions

Men's Health, Rodale

Women's Health, Rodale

Upper Room

Daily Bread

Daily Word

Miracle Cures From The Bible, Reese Dublin

Getting Started On Getting Well, Dr. Lorraine Day, M. D.

Eat To Live, Dr. Joel Fuhrman, M.D.

How I Rebuilt My Immune System After M.S., J.L. Wilson, E.A.